Essential Paediatric MCQs

Essential Paediatric MCQs

Derek I. Johnston
MA MD FRCP DCH
Consultant Paediatrician, University Hospital, Nottingham

David Hull
BSc MB FRCP DObst RCOG DCH
Professor of Child Health, University of Nottingham

THIRD EDITION

CHURCHILL LIVINGSTONE
Medical Division of Pearson Professional Limited

Distributed in the United States of America by Churchill
Livingstone, 650 Avenue of the Americas, New York, N.Y.
10011, and by associated companies, branches and
representatives throughout the world.

First published 1982
Second edition 1989
   Reprinted 1993
   Reprinted 1994
Third edition 1995

ISBN 0-443-05245-X

British Library Cataloguing in Publication Data
A catalog record for this book is available from the British
Library.

Library of Congress Cataloging in Publication Data
A catalogue record for this book is available from the Library
of Congress.

Typeset by Saxon Graphics Ltd, Derby
Produced by Longman Singapore Publishers Pte Ltd
Printed in Singapore

Preface

This collection of MCQs evolved from and complements *Essential Paediatrics*, third edition. There are over one hundred new questions but the format remains as before in that the questions in Chapters 1 to 21 relate to the information provided in the equivalent chapters of *Essential Paediatrics*. The final chapter contains a series of case histories designed to test ability to solve clinical problems and to select appropriate management. The construction of the MCQs follows the formula most widely used in the United Kingdom, a stem followed by five independent items which may be either true or false. Any number of the five items may be correct. The correct answers and an explanation are provided on the page following the questions. A presumed diagnosis is added where this is relevant to the case history.

MCQs are now an inescapable part of the medical student's career. The authors are well aware of their limitations in determining the qualities which make a good doctor but they also see the advantages that they provide in objective assessment. Many of the questions included in this book have been used in undergraduate examinations at Nottingham and all have been reviewed by a panel of clinical teachers. The questions have not, however, been selected solely to provide examination practice. Some are more difficult than will be encountered in the final MB examination, and are appropriate for those preparing for the DCH, but all aim to emphasize important areas in practical paediatrics.

Nottingham, 1995   D.I.J.
                                                                                          D.H.

Contents

1. The ill child and his doctor

1.1 The following reflexes or reactions may be demonstrated in a normal 8-month-old infant
- A Moro reflex
- B stepping reflex
- C parachute reaction
- D palmar grasp reflex
- E traction response

1.2 A 6-week-old infant is normally able to
- A hold his head in the plane of the trunk when pulled by the hands from supine to a sitting position
- B lift his head briefly when placed prone on a flat surface
- C maintain his head in the horizontal plane when held in ventral suspension
- D support his weight on his legs
- E respond to sudden neck extension with asymmetrical arm extension

1.3 A 6-month-old infant is normally able to
- A sit independently for 2 minutes or more
- B play peek-a-boo
- C roll over
- D hold objects with a pincer movement
- E transfer toys from hand to mouth

1.4 A 12-month-old infant can be expected to
- A rise independently from lying to sitting
- B walk alone
- C look for and find objects which roll out of sight
- D pick up crumbs
- E speak six recognizable words

(Answers overleaf)

1.1   C E

The Moro, stepping and palmar grasp reflexes are examples of primary or automatic reactions. They are useful in assessing the functional integrity and maturity of the newborn nervous system. Most are mediated at a subcortical level and are progressively suppressed as normal voluntary motor control evolves. Three months of age represents a watershed at which time the primary reflexes have largely disappeared but have not yet been replaced by postural responses. The Moro reflex becomes progressively less complete after 2 months but may still be elicited up to 5–6 months.

The traction response is demonstrated by pulling the infant by his wrists from the supine to the sitting position. In the neonatal period there is head lag; by 3–4 months the head and trunk are held in a straight line throughout the manoeuvre.

The parachute reaction is a postural response which develops around 7 months. It is elicited by holding the infant around the chest, and moving him suddenly towards the ground in a prone position. A normal response is prompt extension of the limbs as though to break the fall. The test is useful for checking the symmetry of limb movement.

1.2   A B C

The first three tests are all measures of head control and are normally achieved by 6 weeks. Failure may indicate hypotonia due to cerebral pathology, sedation or intercurrent illness.

Voluntary weight bearing does not emerge until 6–8 months.

The Moro response is useful for confirming normal symmetrical arm movement. Failure of an arm to move fully may be due to weakness, fracture or osteomyelitis.

1.3   C E

The 6-month-old sits with minimal support but only momentarily on his own. Rolling over is a complex task and a reliable sign of an intact motor system. He can pick up an object with a palmar grasp as long as both hand and object are in the same visual field. He cannot control release of his grasp so readily until several months older.

He may be friendly to strangers but he is not yet ready to play games.

1.4   A C D

A 12-month-old can normally sit indefinitely, pull to standing and cruise along furniture. He can stand independently only momentarily. He not only looks for dropped objects but deliberately casts them. His vocalization contains most vowel and consonant sounds and he may have up to three words.

1.5 A normal 2 year old should be able to

A climb stairs
B jump from standing position
C pick up a small object such as a raisin with a pincer grasp
D build a tower of 3 bricks
E point to eyes, nose and mouth

1.6 A normal 5 year old should be able to

A consistently catch a tennis ball bounced off the floor
B draw a man with at least 6 parts
C speak fluently and clearly
D participate in sweep audiometry
E write his name

(Answers overleaf)

1.5   **A C D E**
The normal range for walking is up to age 18 months. Two year olds should be able to walk backwards, climb stairs unaided using a hand support, and climb onto a chair. Children may not be acquainted with stairs if they live on one level. Jumping from standing is a more appropriate test for 3 year olds.

The delicate pincer grasp can be used as a test of vision and fine motor function but it also requires mental effort.

Coloured 2.5 cm bricks are invaluable for developmental screening. The child is placed on a parent's lap so as to be able to readily place hands on the table. The tester demonstrates tower building and then offers the bricks one at a time. Building a tower of 3 bricks matches an average of 18 months, and 90% of 2 year olds. By 3.5 years the target is 8 bricks but this may require three attempts.

Pointing to eyes, nose and mouth tests comprehension of speech, and should be achieved by 90% of 2 year olds.

1.6   **B C D**
School entry screening is an important opportunity to detect children with ill-health or developmental problems likely to require special input. Do they have the motor, sensory and social skills necessary to benefit from a hectic environment? Hopefully, most difficulties will have been detected by earlier stages in Child Health Surveillance.

Catching and ball skills are important social attributes but only 50% can reliably catch a tennis ball by age 5 years; 90% should do so by age 6.5 years.

Man or woman drawing has been refined as the Goodenough–Harris Drawing Test with a detailed scoring system dependent on anatomical and clothing accuracy.

Speech assessment is a complex area but as a general rule it should be clear and grammatical by age 4 years.

Sweep audiometry is employed to test groups of children at school entry. Pure-tone audiometry is conducted at 25 dB over the frequency range 250–8000 Hz. Failure in any frequency requires individual evaluation.

1.7 **The following clinical signs in childhood consistently indicate an organic disorder**

    A added sounds on inspiration
    B an apical diastolic murmur
    C an irregular pulse
    D a soft cranial bruit
    E an absent red reflex

1.8 **The following definitions are correct**

    A childhood mortality rate is the number of deaths of children aged 1–14 years in a given year per 100 000 children in this age group
    B infant mortality rate is the number of deaths in infants aged less than 1 year in a given year per 1000 live births
    C perinatal mortality rate is the number of late fetal (24 weeks or more of pregnancy) and early neonatal deaths (infants under 7 days old) in a given year per 1000 total births
    D low birthweight is an infant's weight recorded in the first week of life of below 2500 g
    E prevalence is the number of instances of a given disease or other condition in a given population

1.9 **Over 20% of neonatal deaths are primarily due to**

    A birth trauma
    B birth asphyxia
    C congenital malformation
    D bacterial infection
    E severe immaturity

1.10 **Sudden infant death syndrome has been linked with**

    A adenovirus infection
    B sleep position
    C maternal smoking
    D pertussis immunization
    E overwrapping

1.11 **On hand examination, the following are correct**

    A clinodactyly is the term applied to incurving of the 5th digit
    B single palmar creases are indicative of chromosomal abnormality
    C hypoplasia of the thumb is associated with cardiac lesions
    D nail clubbing does not occur before the second decade
    E narrow nail beds are a feature of Turner syndrome

(Answers overleaf)

1.7   **B E**
In young children transmitted inspiratory noises are often heard over the chest but obviously originate from the upper airway. An apical diastolic murmur must be regarded as implying a significant cardiac lesion, e.g. incompetent semilunar valve or stenosed atrioventricular valve. A diastolic murmur at the base of the heart may be a component of an innocent, extracardiac venous hum and has to be differentiated from the continuous murmur of patent ductus arteriosus.

There are several causes of an innocent irregular pulse in healthy children. Sinus arrhythmia, the variation of heart rate with respiration, may be marked. Extra systoles occur in the absence of underlying disorder; they promptly disappear on exercise.

A soft cranial bruit is not unusual but make a point of auscultating skills as a loud bruit may reveal a pathological arteriovenous shunt. A normal red reflex is an important finding in infancy; it confirms that the ocular light pathway is intact.

1.8   **A B C**
The definitions of mortality rates catch out candidates. We have provided you with the correct versions to avoid any confusion!

Low birthweight means weight at birth or as soon after as is possible.

Prevalence is the number of instances of a given disease or other condition in a given population *at a designated time*.

1.9   **C E**
Congenital malformation and severe prematurity together account for over 80% of neonatal mortality. In 1992 the Nottingham inborn neonatal mortality rate was 5.2 per 1000; this figure falls to 3.9 when infants with lethal malformations are excluded.

1.10   **B C E**
Sudden infant death syndrome (SIDS) describes the unexpected and unexplained death of an apparently healthy infant. This definition depends on there having been an adequate exploration of events before death and an expert postmortem examination. The role of sleep position has emerged as an important issue. Epidemiological studies have highlighted the lower incidence of SIDS in cultures where babies are nursed supine, and the recent decline in UK incidence has paralleled increased public awareness about avoiding prone nursing. Both antenatal and postnatal maternal smoking increase the risk of SIDS. Case-control studies have confirmed that SIDS infants are more likely to be overwrapped. It has been proposed that excessive thermal insulation, possibly combined with a febrile reaction, leads to thermal entrapment.

1.11   **A C E**
This question serves to emphasize the value of close inspection of the hands. Holding a child's hand is also a socially acceptable way of starting the physical examination, after you have accomplished all that can be learned from a distance.

2. Genes

2.1 The following statements are true
A around 5 per 1000 of all liveborn babies have a chromosome abnormality
B a chromosomal abnormality is detectable in less than 10% of spontaneous abortions
C the majority of chromosomal abnormalities arise as an error in gametogenesis in one or other parent
D carriers of a balanced autosomal chromosome rearrangement have a low risk for transmission to offspring
E imbalance of sex chromosomes has more profound mental and physical effects than autosomal imbalance

2.2 Down syndrome
A occurs predominantly among the offspring of mothers aged over 40 years
B is most likely to be due to a chromosome translocation if mother is aged 30 years or younger
C is the most frequent encountered trisomy disorder
D is most frequently due to an isolated meiotic accident
E is significantly less frequent in Asian populations

2.3 Characteristic features of Down syndrome in the newborn include
A hypotonia
B umbilical hernia
C prolonged neonatal jaundice
D single palmar crease
E excess skin on the back of the neck

2.4 A child with Down syndrome is at greater risk from
A duodenal atresia
B meningocele
C deafness
D autoimmune hypothyroidism
E Alzheimer disease

(Answers overleaf)

2.1   **A C**
At least 15% of all recognized pregnancies end in spontaneous miscarriage and in 40% there is a chromosomal abnormality, most commonly autosomal trisomy, monosomy X, triploidy and tetraploidy.

Parents with balanced autosomal rearrangements such as translocation or inversion have a high risk for transmission of an unbalanced form to their children. Loss or gain of autosomal genetic material usually has greater impact on development.

2.2   **C D**
Although increased maternal age is a well established aetiological factor, most Down syndrome children are born to women of normal reproductive age. Non-disjunction, the unequal distribution of 21 group chromatin at fertilization, accounts for 92% of Down syndrome and is much the most common cause at all maternal ages. The remainder are due to sporadic or inherited translocations, and are more likely to be present in younger women. The incidence of 21 trisomy is 1.45 per 1000, and this is constant in different ethnic and socioeconomic groups.

2.3   **A D E**
Hypotonia and excess skin on the back of the neck occur in at least 80% of affected newborns. A single palmar crease is present in 40–50%.

An umbilical hernia and prolonged neonatal jaundice are more in favour of congenital hypothyroidism.

2.4   **A C D E**
Duodenal atresia, anal atresia and congenital heart disease are more frequent in children with Down syndrome. In the recent past the issue of active surgical intervention in potentially handicapped children has challenged paediatricians and their advice to parents. Majority professional opinion and the courts now insist on life-saving procedures unless the complexity and severity of handicap renders such intervention inappropriate.

Both secretory otitis media and sensorineural deafness are more common, and hearing review should be part of the ongoing support offered to these children.

Hypothyroidism is increasingly prevalent after the first decade. It is likely to be overlooked and hence the place for thyroid function tests in routine health screening. Alzheimer disease occurs in the majority by age 40 years.

2.5 Turner syndrome
   A results in spontaneous abortion of the majority of affected fetuses
   B results in failure of differentiation of the Müllerian tube derivatives, i.e. fallopian tubes, uterus and upper vagina
   C is associated with lymphoedema in the newborn
   D results in subnormal intelligence in the typical patient
   E is always associated with pterygium colli (webbing of the neck)

2.6 Characteristic features of Klinefelter syndrome include
   A below average stature
   B hypospadias
   C small testes
   D gynaecomastia
   E mild behavioural disorders

2.7 The following are examples of autosomal dominant inheritance
   A α1-antitrypsin deficiency
   B polyposis coli
   C neurofibromatosis
   D glucose-6-phosphate dehydrogenase deficiency
   E tuberous sclerosis

(Answers overleaf)

2.5   **A C**
It has been calculated that 15% of all pregnancies end in
spontaneous abortion, and that one-tenth of these have the
karyotype 45X. The reason for the high incidence of abortion
among 45X fetuses is unknown.
   The differentiation of the female internal genitalia is
independent of ovarian function. The ovaries appear to undergo
accelerated ageing and become replaced by inactive fibrous
streaks. A minority of these girls, 5–10%, retain sufficient ovarian
function to achieve an abbreviated menarche. For the majority the
low dose oestrogen replacement therapy followed by higher dose
cyclical therapy is the correct strategy for providing puberty.
   It must be remembered that many 45X girls do not have the
florid form. Neck webbing is a feature in about half.

2.6   **C D E**
The typical young man is of average or above average height, the
mean being 2–5 cm above that of the general population. This
reflects genetically determined increased leg length, but is seldom
sufficiently conspicuous to suggest the diagnosis. The penis size
and other secondary sexual characteristics usually fall within the
normal range. The testes are small with severe impairment of
spermatogenesis. Gynaecomastia arises during adolescence in about
half of affected men. It is very variable but may justify cosmetic
reduction procedures. There is a recognized risk of breast cancer.
   Surveys of intelligence show a mild reduction, mean IQ 92.
There is an increased frequency of behavioural problems but
the usual picture is of a rather passive individual with
communication difficulties.

2.7   **B C E**
Polyposis coli or as it is better termed, familial adenomatous
polyposis (FAP), has been referred to as a paediatric blind spot
because it tends to fall within the areas of adult gastroenterology
and genetics! It has a birth prevalence of 1 in 8000, and over
half develop polyps by age 16 years. Malignancy has, however,
been reported as early as age 5 years. FAP is autosomal
dominant and results from loss of the APC gene on
chromosome 5. Molecular genetic analysis now provides for
definite carrier confirmation rather than a 50/50 risk estimate.
   Neurofibromatosis is also a relatively common but highly
variable autosomal dominant disorder with a prevalence of
around 1 in 3000. The classic form with café-au-lait spots,
multiple neurofibromata, iris Lisch nodules and bone lesions is
termed type 1 (NF-1) and has been mapped to chromosome 17.
Type 2 (NF-2) is the variety with familial acoustic neuromas.
   Tuberous sclerosis is a multisystem disorder whose typical
features include the triad of adenoma sebaceum, epilepsy and
mental handicap but there are many variations. It has a
prevalence of between 1 in 10 000 and 1 in 50 000, and as many
as 85% are new mutations. A similar phenotype is produced by
mutations at different sites involving chromosomes 9 and 11.

2.8   The following are examples of autosomal recessive inheritance

A   Huntingdon disease

B   sickle cell disease

C   congenital adrenal hyperplasia

D   spherocytosis

E   myotonic dystrophy

2.9   Features of X-linked recessive inheritance include

A   the absence of biochemical markers of the disorder in carrier women

B   a 1 in 2 risk that a carrier mother will transmit the abnormal gene to a son

C   a 1 in 2 risk that a carrier mother will transmit the abnormal gene to a daughter

D   a 1 in 2 risk that an affected father will transmit the abnormal gene to a son

E   a 1 in 2 risk that an affected father will transmit the abnormal gene to a daughter

2.10   The following disorders have a multifactorial pattern of inheritance

A   cystic fibrosis

B   myelomeningocele

C   Marfan syndrome

D   pyloric stenosis

E   talipes equinovarus

(Answers overleaf)

2.8   **B C**
More than 500 autosomal recessive disorders are recognized
and overall they occur in around 2.5 per 1000 live births. Many
manifest as a biochemical disorder linked to a gene defect of a
specific enzyme pathway, e.g. congenital adrenal hyperplasia
gene defect. The gene responsible for the commonest variety,
21-hydroxylase deficiency, has been mapped to chromosome 6.
  Sickle cell disease is the commonest of the haemoglobinopathies and exemplifies heterozygote advantage with relative
protection in areas endemic for falciparum malaria. The ß-chain
has been mapped to chromosome 11.
  Huntingdon disease, myotonic dystrophy and spherocytosis
are examples of important autosomal dominant, familial
diseases.

2.9   **B C**
It is rare for a woman carrying an X-linked recessive disorder to
have any clinical manifestation. Biochemical tests may be useful
in confirming carrier status, e.g. an elevated serum creatine
kinase level may be detected in around two-thirds of carriers of
Duchenne muscular dystrophy. These indirect measures of gene
activity are now being replaced by direct study of X-linked
genes.
  A carrier mother has a 1 in 2 chance of transmitting the
abnormal gene to a son, who will be affected, or to a daughter,
who will be a carrier.
  An affected male cannot transmit the abnormal X
chromosome to his sons, but he will transmit to all his
daughters who will be carriers.

2.10 **B D E**
Multifactorial inheritance indicates that there are a large number
of both genetic and environmental influences. Surveys of spina
bifida show family aggregations but there is little doubt that
there are potentially preventable environmental factors.
Deficiency of dietary factors, particularly folic acid, is currently
under review. Congenital pyloric stenosis follows a polygenic
model in which the threshold is modified by sex and
environment. As an isolated anomaly, talipes arises from
multifactorial influences.

2.11 The following statements are true

  A   genetic material is transmitted solely via nuclear DNA
  B   approximately 1 per 1000 births carries a dominant gene
      with the potential for handicap
  C   conception in a women of age 45 years introduces a 5%
      chance of chromosome anomaly
  D   cystic fibrosis has been mapped to a single gene locus,
      Δ F508
  E   aneuploidy refers to an alteration of chromosome length

2.12 Fragile X syndrome

  A   is responsible for mental handicap in at least 1 in 1000 males
  B   does not cause mental handicap in carrier females
  C   is associated with autistic behaviour
  D   is associated with enlarged testes
  E   will not be transmitted to the next generation by an
      intellectually normal brother of an affected boy

(Answers overleaf)

2.11   **B C**
DNA is contained within the mitochondria in a double helix closed circular configuration. Mitochondria and their DNA are present in the cytoplasm of the ovum, and hence the transfer of genetic material direct from the mother. This DNA controls fatty acid oxidation and is susceptible to a high rate of mutation which can vary between somatic tissues. The clinical manifestations of the resulting fatty acid oxidation defects are expressed primarily through liver, heart and skeletal muscle.

Mutation of Δ F508 is responsible for about 75% of cystic fibrosis cases but there are at least 150 different mutations accounting for the remaining 25%. Aneuploidy refers to an alteration of chromosome number and is not an exact multiple of the haploid number.

2.12   **A C D**
Fragile X syndrome is the single most commonly recognized form of inherited mental handicap. It has a frequency of 0.3–1 per 1000 males. The disorder results in an IQ in the range 35–50, and may or may not be accompanied by characteristic clinical features such as an elongated face with large ears and prognathism, macro-orchidism after puberty, and mitral valve prolapse. Early signs include language delay and hyperactivity; around 30% meet the criteria of autism.

The fragile X mutation is caused by an unstable region of DNA on the long arm of the X chromosome. This unstable region becomes longer and more unstable with each generation. A critical point is reached when the instability interferes with a brain function determining gene. Although the disorder is usually transmitted in the pattern of sex-linked recessive, there are some unique features. Males carry the mutation but are mentally normal and have a normal chromosome examination. A high proportion of female carriers have mild mental handicap.

3. Fetus

3.1 **The following fetal conditions are associated with raised α–fetoprotein (AFP) levels in maternal blood**
  A   oesophageal atresia
  B   renal agenesis
  C   open neural tube defects
  D   exomphalos
  E   Down syndrome

3.2 **Ultrasonography has an established place in pregnancy to**
  A   assess fetal lung volume
  B   diagnose congenital cardiac disease
  C   determine the velocity of umbilical artery blood flow
  D   establish fetal gender in the first trimester
  E   differentiate gastroschisis from exomphalos

3.3 **Rubella virus infection in the first trimester of pregnancy**
  A   has been eradicated in the UK by current early childhood vaccination programmes
  B   causes a characteristic macular rash in the majority of affected mothers-to-be
  C   causes congenital defects in 15–25% of infants
  D   is a cause of communication disorders in childhood
  E   is a cause of intrauterine growth retardation

(Answers overleaf)

3.1   **A C D**
AFP is the dominant plasma protein in early fetal life prior to the emergence of albumin. Plasma concentrations peak at 3 months and then decline so that it is just detectable at term.

　　Maternal plasma AFP levels at around 16 weeks are elevated in pregnancies with neural tube defects and are used as a screening test. Confirmation can be provided by detailed fetal ultrasound examination. False positive elevated results may be obtained in twin pregnancy, oesophageal atresia and exomphalos. Low levels of AFP correlate with the fetus having Down syndrome, and as part of the triple parameter screening procedure can be used to select mothers for amniocentesis. This combined approach identifies better those mothers at risk across all ages, and has the potential to detect at least twice as many affected fetuses.

3.2   **B C E**
The skilled practitioners of fetal ultrasound have an ever-expanding repertoire, and they provide invaluable assistance in fetal screening and in the definition of suspected abnormality. There are, however, some limitations to their powers of visualization and interpretation.

　　Scans may indicate the shape of the chest but it would be unwise to rely on estimates of lung volume before respiration has commenced. Fetal gender assignment may have important implications for obstetric and later management but genital differentiation and growth is not sufficiently advanced in the first trimester.

3.3   **C D E**
There are two main strategies for the prevention of congenital rubella; the creation of adequate longterm herd immunity by 'universal' early childhood immunization or the selective protection of women of reproductive age. The latter was the policy in the UK until 1988 when the MMR (mumps, measles and rubella) vaccine was introduced for infants of both sexes at age 15 months. Surveys show that not more than half of infected mothers have rashes, and few of these are characteristic.

　　Communication problems, sensorineural deafness and mental handicap are major problems among those who present with manifestations of congenital rubella.

　　Live attenuated rubella virus vaccine is recommended for women of reproductive age with a negative haemagglutination inhibition antibody test. It is contraindicated if the women is or may become pregnant within 2 months. However, the risk of fetal damage following inappropriately timed vaccination has probably been overestimated.

3.4 Cytomegalovirus infection

 A is not a threat to infants of mothers with CMV antibodies
 B may follow viral tranfer via breast milk
 C is a cause of microcephaly
 D merits routine screening of all pregnancies
 E during fetal life results in recognizable symptoms in over half
    of the resulting children

3.5 Polyhydramnios has a recognized association with

 A fetal upper gastrointestinal tract obstruction
 B severe rhesus isoimmunization
 C renal agenesis
 D trisomy disorders
 E pulmonary hypoplasia

3.6 Symmetrical fetal growth retardation is associated with

 A intrauterine infection
 B fetal alcohol syndrome
 C congenital hypothyroidism
 D chromosomal abnormality
 E third trimester utero-placental failure

(Answers overleaf)

3.4   **B C**
Cytomegalovirus is probably the most common congenital
infection in developed countries, and is an important cause of
mental and sensory handicap. The proportion of children and
adults who acquire CMV antibody varies with geographical and
socioeconomic status. It is estimated that 50–60% of pregnant
women in the UK already have antibody; this does not provide
complete protection against reinfection or reactivation. Between
1 and 6% of pregnant women in the UK excrete virus and
congenital transmission to the fetus occurs in 0.3–0.4%. A
higher percentage of infants are infected postnatally, commonly
via breast milk. Postnatal infection is usually asymptomatic but
that arising from blood transfusion to very low birthweight
infants can result in significant morbidity.

Ninety per cent of congenitally infected infants remain free of
symptoms; about 2% develop neurological handicap. We are
not yet equipped with either protective vaccine or antiviral
agents, and routine screening has no place.

3.5   **A B D**
Polyhydramnios refers to a clinical estimate of amniotic fluid
volume in excess of 2 litres. The fluid accumulates if the fetus
has a neurological or anatomical disorder preventing swallowing
and absorption. The paediatrician must be alert to the latter and
prepared to pass a wide-bore orogastric tube. Other causes
include poorly controlled maternal diabetes, severe umbilical
cord compression and a variety of fetal malformations.

3.6   **A B D**
Symmetrical growth retardation describes the infant in whom
the three main parameters of growth: head circumference,
length and weight are all subnormal for gestation. It reflects
either an intrinsic cause of growth failure, e.g. a genetic defect,
or an external restraint imposed from early to mid pregnancy,
e.g. congenital rubella or excessive alcohol exposure. This
pattern is likely to determine permanent small stature. By
contrast, late pregnancy utero-placental failure primarily reduces
body size leaving head growth protected. The resultant newborn
infant usually exhibits rapid catch-up growth.

Infants with congenital hypothyroidism are often delivered
post-term and with above average birth size.

3.7   The following are recognized associations

A   maternal intravenous glucose infusion and neonatal hyponatraemia

B   maternal heroin addiction and a reduced incidence of respiratory distress syndrome

C   maternal heparin therapy and neonatal intracranial haemorrhage

D   maternal carbimazole and fetal goitre

E   maternal insulin and fetal hypoglycaemia

3.8   The following organisms, if present in the birth canal, place the newborn full-term infant at increased risk of systemic infection

A   *Candida albicans*

B   Herpes simplex

C   Group B streptococcus

D   *Trichomonas vaginalis*

E   *Chlamydia trachomatis*

(Answers overleaf)

3.7   **A B D E**
Drugs should be prescribed in pregnancy only if the benefit to
the mother is considered to outweigh the potential for risk to the
fetus. Drugs should be avoided in the first trimester when the
risk of teratogenesis is greatest but care is needed throughout
pregnancy. *The British National Formulary* contains a detailed
appendix devoted to prescribing in pregnancy.

Even apparently innocent drugs or intravenous fluid
administration in the perinatal period may have adverse effects
on the neonate. Liberal use of intravenous glucose infusion has
been linked to neonatal hyponatraemia and convulsions.

Heroin cannot be recommended to reduce the incidence of
respiratory distress syndrome but it is a well documented effect!

Neither heparin nor insulin crosses the placenta to any extent;
however, maternal hypoglycaemia results in a net drain on fetal
glucose and hence hypoglycaemia.

3.8   **B C E**
Neonatal herpes infection is a relatively rare but life-threatening
illness. The main route of infection is by intrapartum contact
with maternal herpes but in 60–80% of cases the mothers have
neither a history of genital herpes nor any evidence of active
lesions. This reduces the place for antenatal screening and there
is no need for asymptomatic women, with only a history of
herpes, to be subjected to caesarian section.

Group B streptococcus acquired from the birth canal is a key
cause of early onset pneumonia, septicaemia and meningitis.
Infection may resemble severe birth asphyxia, and it needs to be
considered in preterm infants with respiratory distress. It
appears to be less common in Europe, 0.16–0.3 per 1000,
compared to the US, 3.7 per 1000. *Chlamydia trachomatis* is
commonly associated with neonatal conjunctivitis and it may
produce pneumonia. It has also been linked to fetal pneumonia
and an early neonatal septicaemic-like illness.

Candida infection is common but seldom invasive in
otherwise healthy infants.

3.9 The following are recognized approaches to fetal therapy

A maternal carbimazole therapy in fetal thyrotoxicosis

B maternal phenobarbitone therapy in fetal cholestasis

C maternal thyroid therapy in congenital hypothyroidism

D maternal dexamethasone therapy in fetal 21-hydroxylase deficiency

E maternal digoxin therapy in fetal supraventricular tachycardia

3.10 A full-term normal infant

A has a serum IgG concentration equivalent to about 20% of adult levels

B will respond to infection by increased production of IgM

C will absorb IgG from human breast milk

D will absorb IgA from human breast milk

E is equipped with active cellular immunity

(Answers overleaf)

3.9   **A D E**

Fetal medicine is a rapidly growing field fostered by close liaison between obstetricians, equipped with the means for examining the intrauterine patient, and paediatricians promoting optimal care for immature and sick infants. Some of the more interventional procedures are pioneering and require validation. Other medical management exploiting drug transfer across the placenta is well-established.

Fetal thyrotoxicosis is a potential hazard in the 0.5–2 per 1000 pregnancies in which the mother has thyroid stimulating antibodies. Fetal tachycardia may be a prodrome to stillbirth, and can be controlled by administering carbimazole to the mother who may also require thyroxine to maintain her euthyroid. Thyroxine does not cross the placenta to any extent.

It is possible to reduce the severity of virilization in female fetuses affected by 21-hydroxylase deficiency (congenital adrenal hyperplasia) by administering dexamethasone to mothers in early pregnancy. This strategy requires counselling and preparation before pregnancy.

Fetal supraventricular tachycardia needs to be considered in the differential diagnosis of sudden onset or intermittent fetal tachycardia and distress.

3.10   **B E**

Fetal serum IgG levels are of the same order as those in the maternal circulation. The infant's immune defence systems are well developed at birth but relatively untested. The benefit, if any, that the infant gains from breast milk immunoglobulins remains unproven. There is no evidence to suggest that the human infant, like the newborn pig, gains much IgG from milk.

4. Newborn

4.1 Newborn infants commonly have
- A a capillary haemangioma on the forehead
- B a posterior cranial fontanelle
- C a metopic suture
- D impalpable coronal sutures
- E skin tags in front of the ear

4.2 Newborn infants commonly have
- A papulovesicles over the trunk
- B posterior fusion of the labia minora
- C an adherent foreskin
- D breast enlargement
- E a shallow sacral dimple

4.3 Birth injury accounts for the majority of the following conditions detected in early infancy
- A intraventricular haemorrhage
- B cephalohaematoma
- C hydrocephalus
- D facial nerve palsy
- E pneumothorax

4.4 Two minutes after a normal term delivery
- A the ductus venosus will be closed
- B the pulmonary arterial pressure will have fallen
- C the pressure in the left atrium will have fallen
- D the arterial oxygen tension will have risen
- E regular breathing will have begun

(Answers overleaf)

4.1   A B C
Flame haemangiomas are common on the bridge of the nose, forehead and eyelids, and are invariably matched by those on the nape of the neck. The normal skull has six fontanelles; anterior, posterior, two sphenoid and two mastoid. The posterior fontanelle usually closes by 2 months but may be impalpable at birth. Absent sutures are as significant as abnormally wide ones. Preauricular skin tags raise the suspicion of first branchial arch malformations and deafness.

4.2   A C D E
Crops of papules, miliaria, are common and reflect sweat gland immaturity. Clitoromegally and labial prominence can cause concern particularly in small-for-dates infants, but the absence of labial fusion helps to rule out virilization.

4.3   B D
Birth trauma may result in extra- or intracranial damage. Tentorial tears are generally limited to full-term infants delivered through too small a birth canal, or to premature infants with compliant skulls. Fortunately, the majority of subdural haemorrhages are small and clinically insignificant. Intra- or periventricular haemorrhages reflect the inability of the very immature vasculature of this region to tolerate abrupt alterations of perfusion. Hydrocephalus may arise from congenital malformation or infection, or from an acquired disorder, intracranial haemorrhage or infection.
   The majority of facial nerve palsies are caused by compression of the nerve against the ramus of the mandible during forceps delivery. They usually recover over days or weeks.

4.4   A B D E
When the umbilical cord is clamped the blood flow returning from the placenta ceases suddenly and the ductus venosus closes. As a consequence the pressure in the *right* atrium falls. As the baby cries and expands the lungs the pulmonary vascular bed opens and the pulmonary arterial pressure falls. With expansion of the lungs the arterial oxygen tension rises. All this usually happens within the first 2 minutes of life.

4.5 Established neonatal resuscitation procedures include
A directing a cold stream of oxygen at the nose
B administration of drugs with respiratory stimulant properties
C oropharyngeal suction
D bag and face-mask ventilation
E prompt cooling

4.6 The Apgar score
A at 1 minute is a reliable measure of asphyxia
B at 1 minute is a useful measure of respiratory failure
C at 10 minutes is strongly correlated with later neurological deficit
D includes the infant's response to a pharyngeal suction catheter
E is not applicable after 10 minutes of age

4.7 A newborn infant who remains centrally cyanosed after intubation and intermittent positive pressure ventilation may have
A a diaphragmatic hernia
B choanal atresia
C a tension pneumothorax
D drug-induced respiratory centre impairment
E profound anaemia

4.8 A preterm infant is at increased risk from
A conjugated hyperbilirubinaemia
B meconium aspiration
C periventricular leucomalacia
D necrotizing enterocolitis
E child abuse

(Answers overleaf)

4.5   **A C D**
Facial oxygen is one of several gentle, harmless peripheral stimuli which may be all that are needed to provoke adequate spontaneous ventilation. Oropharyngeal suction is important when there is an appropriate indication, such as the upper airway containing blood, meconium or other extraneous liquid. It is not justified as a mere routine to remove the clear fluid of pulmonary origin that transiently appears in the oropharynx. Bag and mask ventilation, using correct equipment and technique, can be effective as a temporary measure until adequate ventilation is established. A poor response after 4–5 minutes (or earlier in low birthweight infants) demands tracheal intubation and intermittent positive pressure ventilation.

The use of respiratory stimulants is physiologically unsound and potentially dangerous. Naloxone is not a respiratory stimulant but is given to reverse the depressive effect of maternal opiates. It should be administered only after respiration has been established. Cooling has to be actively avoided, not promoted!

4.6   **B C D**
The Apgar scoring system is a widely accepted shorthand for summarizing the status of the newborn. In the first minutes it highlights infants who require active resuscitation. It is, however, a clinical assessment based on observation during a brief timespan, and correlates poorly with asphyxia, which may have originated long before delivery. Later scores, performed after effective resuscitation, are far better guides to prognosis.

4.7   **A C**
The first priority is to exclude technical errors, e.g. faulty insertion of the endotracheal tube. If resuscitation has been appropriate the infant is likely to have a severe structural problem of the lungs or heart. Choanal atresia comes to light when the infant repeatedly becomes apnoeic on removing the endotracheal tube, but is otherwise vigorous.

4.8   **C D E**
Periventricular leucomalacia reflects the parenchymal damage produced by ischaemia and has a higher correlation with neurodevelopmental disability than haemorrhage alone. The early ischaemic lesions produce a flare on cerebral ultrasound which may appear to resolve or may progress to cystic change.

Necrotizing enterocolitis (NEC) is a serious gastrointestinal disease of preterm infants. It carries a substantial morbidity from gut perforation, obstruction, short bowel syndrome and secondary liver disease as well as contributing to mortality. It also complicates neonatal nutrition programmes and adds to duration of intensive care and cost. The precise causes remain elusive although breast milk feeding appears to be protective.

Non-accidental injury is more common in this group. This may reflect adverse socioeconomic factors and the higher prevalence of very young mothers of low birthweight infants. We also need to recognize the disruption to bonding and family life produced by prolonged admission to neonatal units.

4.9   Peri- or intraventricular cerebral haemorrhage
A   occurs in less than 10% of very low birthweight infants
B   arises most commonly in the first 72 hours after delivery
C   is a direct result of impaired vitamin K supply
D   is the single most common cause of congenital cerebral palsy
E   may result in rapidly evolving hydrocephalus

4.10   A full-term small-for-dates infant is at increased risk from
A   meconium aspiration
B   hyperbilirubinaemia
C   feeding problems
D   hypothermia
E   associated congenital anomalies

4.11   Infants of diabetic mothers are at increased risk from
A   hypocalcaemia
B   anaemia
C   jaundice
D   shoulder dystocia
E   congenital abnormalities

4.12   Respiratory distress in newborn babies is a recognized complication of
A   group B streptococcal infection
B   congenital heart disease
C   sickle cell disease
D   cerebral disorders
E   diaphragmatic hernia

(Answers overleaf)

4.9   **B E**
As many as 50% of infants of birthweight less than 1500 g have
evidence of periventricular haemorrhage on ultrasound
examination. The responsible mechanism has yet to be defined,
but is thought to involve the fragility of the rich vascular network
which lies adjacent to the lateral ventricles. Stresses imposed by
hypoxia, hypotension and acidaemia aggravate the vessel
fragility. There are no readily correctable coagulation disorders.
   The majority of affected infants escape detectable longterm
neurodevelopmental sequelae. Those with extensive haemorrhages
and associated ischaemic damage are likely to develop mental
handicap, cerebral palsy, hydrocephalus and seizures.
Epidemiological studies reveal that prematurity contributes a
minority of cases of cerebral palsy. A study in North East England
showed that infants with a birthweight of 2500 g or greater
accounted for two-thirds of cases of congenital cerebral palsy.

4.10 **A D E**
Small-for-dates infants are potentially at risk in late pregnancy
and during delivery. They tolerate hypoxia poorly and a feature
of their distress is the passage of meconium with the resultant
hazard of inhalation and pneumonia. It is rare for a preterm
infant to pass meconium in utero.
   The large relative surface area and low fat reserves of these
infants make them vulnerable to hypothermia.
   Symmetrical low birthweight, that is small head size as well as
body size, raises the possibility of an intrinsic growth restraint.
Congenital abnormality needs to be excluded by careful physical
examination and there is a low threshold for ultrasound imaging
and chromosome analysis.

4.11 **A C D E**
Polycythaemia is more probable than anaemia. Improved
control of maternal diabetes has diminished the previously
important hazards of relative immaturity, excessive size and
metabolic derangement. There continues to be a three to
fourfold increased rate of congenital malformation in these
infants. This can be lowered by achieving optimal metabolic
control prior to conception and by maintaining it during the
phase of fetal organogenesis.

4.12 **A B D E**
Respiratory distress is not always due to airway or lung disease.
Septicaemia, cerebral lesions, heart disease and metabolic
acidosis enter the differential diagnosis. The premature infant
with group B streptococcal infection may be in a poor condition
at birth or present after a few hours with grunting and
recession: a pattern initially indistinguishable from idiopathic
respiratory distress syndrome.

4.13   Clinical jaundice in the first week of life

A   occurs in less than 10% of full-term infants
B   is normally associated with unconjugated hyperbilirubinaemia
C   is commoner after breech delivery
D   is increased in association with the early passage of meconium
E   is a feature of congenital infection

4.14   Features typical of physiological jaundice include

A   recognizable jaundice in the first 48 hours
B   peak plasma bilirubin at 4–5 days
C   persistence beyond first week
D   irritability
E   pale stools

4.15   A newborn infant may present with bile-stained vomiting and abdominal distension as the result of

A   oesophageal atresia
B   duodenal atresia
C   birth asphyxia
D   electrolyte disturbance
E   cystic fibrosis

4.16   The following features are consistent with a newborn infant having oesophageal atresia and a tracheo-oesophageal fistula

A   maternal polyhydramnios
B   passage of a wide-bore orogastric catheter into the stomach
C   plain X-ray evidence of air in the stomach and small bowel
D   plain X-ray evidence of hemivertebrae
E   excessive mucus in the nostrils or mouth

(Answers overleaf)

4.13   B C E
Up to 50% of healthy newborn infants become recognizably
jaundiced. The great majority have so-called physiological
jaundice, reflecting the breakdown of haem at a time of hepatic
immaturity and before full milk intake has been established.
Breech and forceps deliveries are liable to produce extensive
bruising which adds to the load of haem and hence
unconjugated bilirubin. The delayed passage of meconium may
signal the presence of intestinal obstruction with accompanying
problems of reduced nutrient intake and increased bilirubin
reabsorption.

4.14   B
Staff caring for newborn infants must be vigilant for features
which vary from the typical pattern of physiological jaundice.
Jaundice detected in the first 48 hours should be regarded as
being due to abnormal haemolysis until proved otherwise.
Persistence beyond 7 days, end even up to 2–3 weeks, may be
innocent, particularly in premature or breastfed infants.
However, persistent jaundice is not typical and affected babies
require at least regular observation, checking for features that
might suggest an underlying disorder. Pale stools, a cardinal
sign of cholestasis, do not receive the interest they deserve.

4.15   B C D E
Small bowel obstruction may arise as the result of functional
ileus linked to respiratory disorders, asphyxia, hypokalaemia and
infection. Delayed passage of meconium, absence of systemic
problems and features on plain abdominal X-ray usually confirm
anatomical obstruction. In duodenal obstruction, the atretic
segment is distal to the sphincter of Oddi and hence the
production of bile-stained vomit. Between 10 and 20% of infants
with cystic fibrosis present with meconium ileus.

4.16   A C D E
It is essential to diagnose oesophageal atresia promptly and
before the first attempt at feeding. All infants with maternal
polyhydramnios should be checked by the passage of a wide-
bore, size 10 or diameter 6–7 mm, orogastric catheter. A finer
catheter may coil in the oesophageal pouch giving the false
impression of continuity, or take a devious route through the
upper trachea and fistula to reach the lower oesophagus and
stomach. Inability to pass a wide-bore catheter needs to be
checked with antero-posterior and lateral X-rays.
    Oesophageal atresia is commonly associated with other
anomalies in the gastrointestinal (duodenal and anorectal
atresia), urinary, cardiac and skeletal systems.

4.17   Vitamin K

    A is an essential cofactor for the synthesis of coagulation factors II, VII, IX and X

    B is readily transported across the placenta

    C is present in breast milk at a higher concentration than in cow's milk

    D given in a single oral dose after delivery effectively prevents haemorrhagic disease

    E related haemorrhage in the newborn is commoner when mothers have taken anticonvulsants during pregnancy

4.18   The following are recognized causes of neonatal convulsions

    A birth asphyxia

    B hypoglycaemia

    C hypothermia

    D opiate withdrawal

    E hypernatraemia

4.19   Intrauterine posture is commonly responsible for

    A congenital dislocation of the hip

    B plagiocephaly

    C sternomastoid shortening

    D syndactyly

    E mandibular asymmetry

(Answers overleaf)

4.17   **A   E**
National strategies for the prevention of haemorrhagic disease of the newborn have recently come under review. There has been a move away from universal intramuscular vitamin K administration at delivery to the use of oral preparations. Unfortunately, single doses of oral vitamin K given on day 1 do not provide complete protection, particularly in breastfed infants or in those with underlying liver disease. Human milk is relatively low in vitamin K (2 µg/l) compared to cow's milk (4–18 µg/l). Vitamin K absorption is dependent on intact bile flow and pancreatic function so that infants with neonatal cholestasis or malabsorption are also at increased risk. Revised national guidelines promote oral administration at delivery followed by repeat oral doses in breastfed infants.
Drugs which interfere with vitamin K metabolism include phenytoin, warfarin, rifampicin and isoniazid. Infants of mothers taking these drugs are at increased risk of early severe haemorrhagic disease. One preventative measure is to give the mother high dose vitamin K before delivery. Placental transport of vitamin K is limited and hence the requirement for high doses.

4.18   **A   B   D   E**
The maternal and birth histories are important in providing clues to existence of birth asphyxia, hypoxic–ischaemic encephalopathy, or the risk of drug withdrawal. Several causes may be superimposed and hence the place for an investigative scheme including blood glucose, calcium and electrolytes, as well as an infection screen and a brain ultrasound.

4.19   **A   B   C   E**
Persisting deformities may arise when fetal mobility is restricted, most commonly because of reduced amniotic fluid volume. Congenital dislocation of the hip has a multifactorial aetiology but an important component is intrauterine position, notably breech presentation. Plagiocephaly refers to skull asymmetry in which one hemicranium is positioned anteriorly compared to the other so that half the forehead is more prominent and the ipsilateral occiput is flattened. Persistence after the first weeks of life may reflect an associated reduction of neck mobility due to sternomastoid shortening. Mandibular asymmetry is a further component of this deformation group. These deformities usually correct spontaneously in a normally mobile infant. Simple exercises guided by a paediatric physiotherapist hasten improvement in more severe cases.
Syndactyly or fusion of digits are relatively common inherited malformations. Most are isolated and have a dominant pattern of inheritance. They may however be a marker of more generalized syndromes.

4.20 Established neonatal screening tests include
    A umbilical cord blood analysis to detect phenylketonuria
    B umbilical cord blood analysis to detect galactose
    C umbilical cord blood analysis to detect sickle cell disease
    D capillary blood analysis at 6–8 days to detect elevated TSH
    E capillary blood analysis at 6–8 days to detect elevated
       immunoreactive trypsin

(Answer overleaf)

4.20 **C D E**
There is constant pressure to increase the range of disorders
encompassed by neonatal blood test screening. However, not
all the bids meet the WHO criteria of a condition which should
be an important public health problem, have a natural history
which is adequately understood, and have an agreed strategy
for diagnosis and treatment.
  Phenylketonuria (1 in 10 000 live births) is diagnosed by the
measurement of blood phenylalanine, e.g. the Guthrie inhibition
technique, at age 6–8 days by which time the infant should be
established on milk.
  Galactosaemia (1 in 70 000 live births) is not screened for
routinely, not only because it is very rare but because clinical
presentation is usually early and before potential screening of
6–8-day capillary blood would reveal it. There is negligible
endogenous synthesis of galactose and hence no place for
measuring blood or urinary galactose before milk intake. In
situations where the clinical picture or family history suggest
galactosaemia, the preferred test is direct enzyme assay of
galactose-1-phosphate uridyl transferase in red blood cells.
  In selected populations, sickle cell disease (SS disease) is as
common as 1 in 300 births. Since much of its morbidity occurs
in the first 3 years of life, early diagnosis is valuable in order to
implement prophylactic programmes.
  The detection of congenital hypothyroidism (1 in 3500 live
births) and the prevention of mental handicap is one of the great
success stories of screening programmes.
  Cystic fibrosis (1 in 2500 live births) is being screened for by
detection of elevated immunoreactive trypsin levels.
Unfortunately, this method has poor specificity and is raised in 1
in 200 tests. Specificity can be increased by further analysing
DNA from the initial sample for the Δ F508 mutation.

5. Nutrition

5.1   Vitamin D deficiency
 A   causes limb pain
 B   causes muscle weakness
 C   is usually confirmed by finding a subnormal plasma calcium level
 D   results in a depressed plasma phosphate level
 E   is prevented by the provision of free school milk

5.2   Breast milk
 A   contains sucrose
 B   contains a large proportion of protein as whey
 C   contains the majority of fat as medium chain triglycerides
 D   promotes the growth of bifidobacteria in the gut
 E   contains macrophages

5.3   The following nutritional advice is correct
 A   hungry bottle-fed babies should be converted from a whey-based to a casein-based formula
 B   unmodified cow's milk is nutritionally appropriate for infants from age 3 months
 C   weaning should be started between age 3 and 6 months
 D   vitamin drops are recommended from age 6 months until at least 2 years
 E   goat's milk is indicated in children with cow's milk intolerance

(Answers overleaf)

5.1   **A B D**
Limb pain, irritability and muscle weakness are features of
vitamin D deficiency. The latter contributes to delayed standing
and walking. The biochemical markers are a raised alkaline
phosphatase level and a depressed phosphate concentration.
Skeletal calcium is mobilized to maintain normocalcaemia.
   The low vitamin D content of cow's milk is unlikely to prevent
the evolution of rickets. Exposure to sunlight in the playground
is more important!

5.2   **B D E**
The majority of milk carbohydrate is in the form of the
disaccharide lactose, a compound of glucose and galactose.
   The faecal flora of breastfed babies is dominated by
commensals such as bifidobacteria. By contrast, bottlefed
babies are colonized by potential pathogens such as *Escherichia
coli*. Numerous breast milk constituents are responsible for the
pattern of gut flora, e.g. lactoferrin.
   Fresh breast milk is a biologically active solution containing
both cellular and humoral immune agents as well as endocrine
factors.

5.3   **C D**
Whey-based formulae have a whey/casein ratio similar to
human milk, that is 60/40. Casein-based formulae contain a ratio
of 20/80 matching cow's milk. The casein milks are promoted as
being more satisfying with benefit to sleep pattern and growth.
There is no evidence to support this advice, and mothers report
benefits from transferring in either direction.
   Although the introduction of solids is reasonable from age 3
months, it is not actively promoted until age 6 months. It is
preferable to continue breast or infant formulae until 12 months.
Cow's milk is high in protein and low in iron.
   Vitamin deficiency is rare with conventional feeding practices
in Europe. Nevertheless, current Department of Health
recommendations include the use of vitamin drops for this age
group, partly as a safety net to provide for infants subjected to
delayed weaning, deprivation or restricted diets.
   Goat and sheep milk should not be used for human infant
nutrition because the solute load is high and the mineral and
vitamin (particularly folate) content unsuitable.

5.4   **Breast milk**

A   fed to preterm infants increases neurodevelopmental scores
    in later childhood
B   is protective against infection during infancy
C   results in lower serum cholesterol levels
D   is protective against sudden infant death syndrome
E   is protective against haemorrhagic disease of the newborn

5.5   In comparison with breast milk, cow's milk contains
A   more calcium
B   more lactose
C   more sodium
D   a higher curd/whey ratio
E   more unsaturated fat

5.6   Gastro-oesophageal reflux enters into the differential diagnosis of
A   recurrent pneumonia
B   'near miss cot death'
C   abnormal neck posturing
D   hypochromic, microcytic anaemia
E   failure to thrive

5.7   Pyloric stenosis
A   is due to thickening of the circular muscle fibres of the
    pylorus
B   is inherited by a sex-linked pattern
C   presents most commonly at 8–12 weeks of age
D   results in bile-stained vomits
E   results in metabolic acidosis

5.4   A   B   D

(Answers overleaf)

Prospective studies have shown that donor breast milk given to preterm infants during the first month of life has a beneficial impact on neurodevelopmental scores at 18 months corrected age. Nutrient-enriched formulae also benefit the development of preterm infants but there are probably factors independent of energy content in breast milk. Candidate substances are long-chain ω-6 and ω-3 fatty acids, e.g. arachidonic and docosahexanoic acid, which are found in abundance in brain and retina.

Breast milk and especially colostrum contains important anti-infective properties. Maternal secretory IgA and IgM are conditioned by the enteromammary and bronchomammary axes to be specific against antigens in the environment. The concentration of immunocompetent cells is also high.

Haemorrhagic disease of the newborn occurs in approximately 8 per 100 000 live births and is more frequent in breastfed infants. The late variety is associated with a 50% risk of an intracranial bleed. These figures provide a compelling case for routine vitamin K prophylaxis either by intramuscular injection or by a 3 or 4 dose oral regimen.

5.5   **A C D**
Cow's milk does contain more calcium, but also more phosphorus and it is the latter which is partly responsible for the calcium not being absorbed and thus leaving the infant at risk of hypocalcaemia. Cow's milk also contains more sodium; concentrated feeds can cause dangerous hypernatraemia. Curds in cow's milk make it more difficult to digest. The bacteria in animals with multiple stomachs saturate unsaturated fatty acids and reduce the content of essential fatty acids.

5.6   **A B C D E**
Mild gastro-oesophageal reflux is a common occurrence in early infancy. In its more severe forms it can manifest as any of the above problems. Aspiration may be responsible for persistent chest problems, or, more acutely, may provoke obstructive apnoea and the threat of sudden infant death syndrome. Painful oesophagitis may cause the child to adopt unusual neck posturing. This can be confused with seizures, especially when it is exhibited by a handicapped child otherwise unable to voice his discomfort.

5.7   **A**
Although pyloric stenosis is commoner in males, it is inherited by the polygenic mode. There are also, as yet unidentified, environmental factors to which the male appears more susceptible. The peak incidence occurs in the first 4–6 weeks of life; premature infants may develop the problem before their expected date of birth. The loss of gastric secretions results in metabolic alkalosis. Metabolic acidosis is incompatible with this diagnosis and raises the possibility of infection, renal failure, adrenal failure or an inborn error of metabolism.

5.8   **Three month colic**

A   is an indication for a trial of soya protein-based milk formula
B   is an indication for the early introduction of a weaning diet
C   is typically accompanied by the infant becoming flushed
D   is associated with feed refusal
E   is an indication for dicyclomine hydrochloride

5.9   Dental caries

A   is caused by *Streptococcus viridans*
B   is the result of acid attack on enamel
C   is less likely in fissures
D   is less common in children with insulin-dependent diabetes
E   is commoner in children with epilepsy

5.10   The following are good sources of iron

A   cow's milk
B   chicken
C   cereals
D   brussel sprouts
E   fish

5.11   The brain

A   accounts for approximately 10% of total body weight at birth
B   accounts for approximately 10% of total body weight at 1 year
C   utilizes approximately 10% of total energy intake during the first year
D   neuronal membranes contain high concentrations of polyunsaturated fatty acids
E   has largely completed myelination by 40 weeks gestation

5.8   C

(Answers overleaf)

A pattern of evening fussing and apparent colicky discomfort affects up to 40% of infants between 3 weeks and 3 months. Apart from features suggesting increased gastrointestinal motility, we know little of its aetiology. Occasional infants have evidence of either milk allergy or lactose intolerance but it is inappropriate to make radical alterations to feeding regimens for the majority of affected babies. Simple guidance and reassurance are usually sufficient. Feed refusal favours more specific pathology, e.g. urinary tract infection. Antispasmodics, particularly dicyclomine, have been widely prescribed in the past but are no longer recommended under age 6 months.

5.9   A B D E
Dental caries remains a priority in child health although the proportion of 5 year olds in England and Wales with recognized tooth decay fell from 71% in 1973 to 48% in 1983. Most sugars serve as a substrate for oral streptococci, and result in the creation of lactic acid and plaque. The acid damages enamel, and the plaque provides the bacteria with a protective shield. Caries is commoner in fissures. It is also more prevalent in children maintained on longterm syrup-based medication.

5.10   B D
Prolonged milk feeding without adequate introduction of a mixed diet is a common cause of iron deficiency.

5.11   A B D
There are still important unresolved issues in the optimal design of infant formulae. Brain development, and in particular the fatty acid composition of neuronal membranes, is an area where nutrition may influence neurodevelopmental performance. The brain accounts for 60% of total energy intake in the first year, and polyunsaturated fatty acids (PUFAs) are an essential ingredient of neuronal myelination. Human milk contains readily synthesized PUFAs, especially docohexanoic and arachidonic acid. Infant formulae contain little if any PUFAs but should include sufficient of the precursor essential fatty acids, linoleic acid and α-linolenic acid.

6. Infection

6.1 **The following are components of the UK National Immunization Schedule**

    A   three doses of diptheria/tetanus/pertussis (DTP) and polio by age 6 months

    B   one dose of Hib by age 6 months

    C   measles/mumps/rubella (MMR) by age 15 months

    D   booster diptheria/tetanus and polio by 5 years

    E   booster measles/mumps/rubella (MMR) at age 4–5 years

6.2 **Rubella**

    A   has an incubation of 14–21 days

    B   commonly results in a temperature above 38°C

    C   is typically accompanied by posterior cervical lymphadenopathy

    D   is associated with thrombocytopenic purpura

    E   can be readily identified on the basis of its characteristic rash

6.3 **Chicken pox**

    A   is caused by the same virus that causes herpes zoster

    B   presents with vesicles mainly on the arms and legs

    C   rarely causes lesions in the mouth

    D   may be complicated by cerebellar ataxia

    E   should be treated with an immunoglobulin injection in immune deficient individuals

6.4 **Herpes simplex infection**

    A   is usually benign when acquired at birth

    B   commonly causes acute gingivostomatitis

    C   is a cause of paronychia

    D   is a cause of keratoconjunctivitis

    E   is the most common sporadic cause of encephalitis

(Answers overleaf)

6.1   **A C D**
DTP and polio plus Hib make up the primary immunization course given as three injections at 2, 3 and 4 months (or to be completed by 6 months with intervals between injections of not less than 1 month).
MMR is recommended before age 15 months and should be given irrespective of a history of measles, mumps and rubella. MMR may be given at any age but reimmunization is not recommended.

6.2   **A C D**
Rubella is typically mild with a low-grade fever and an often transient, diffuse maculopapular rash. The rash is by no means characteristic but the accompanying suboccipital lymph node enlargement may help clinical recognition. Complications in children are few and usually mild; arthritis, encephalitis and thrombocytopenia.

6.3   **A D E**
Chicken pox spots appear as crops, mainly over the trunk. Oral ulcers can be troublesome. Children with immune deficiency, including those receiving antileukaemic therapy, must be provided with zoster-immune globulin if exposure is suspected.

6.4   **B C D E**
Active Herpes simplex infection of the mother's genital tract is potentially a serious threat to her infant. Maternal antibodies may not be protective if the current infection is due to a new strain of virus. The majority of children have relatively benign manifestations of primary infection. The virus is readily spread by direct contact, particularly to damaged skin, and hence secondary involvement of sucked fingers or eczematous skin patches.
The enteroviruses (Coxsachie, polio and Echo virus) are commoner infective agents in seasonally related outbreaks, but Herpes simplex is the commonest identified sporadic cause.

6.5   Mumps

   A   is caused by an enterovirus
   B   is commonly manifest by a mild non-specific illness
   C   is the predominant cause of acute parotitis
   D   rarely results in cerebrospinal fluid pleocytosis
   E   is a cause of sensorineural deafness

6.6   Glandular fever (infectious mononucleosis)

   A   is caused by Epstein-Barr virus
   B   is the sole cause of a positive Monospot test
   C   causes an exudative tonsillitis
   D   is rare in preschool children
   E   causes transient immunodeficiency

6.7   Pertussis (whooping cough)

   A   seldom occurs in the first 3 months of life
   B   typically commences with a catarrhal phase
   C   is associated with a reduced blood lymphocyte count
   D   is abbreviated following treatment with erythromycin
   E   is a cause of persistent vomiting

6.8   Tuberculosis in early childhood

   A   is most frequently initiated by a primary focus in the gut
   B   carries a high risk of extrapulmonary involvement
   C   seldom results in haemoptysis
   D   is consistently associated with a positive tuberculin reaction
   E   necessitates admission to isolation facilities

(Answers overleaf)

6.5   **B C E**
Mumps is caused by a paramyxovirus. Approximately half of
infected children have minimal illness. Acute parotitis is
characteristic of mumps but may occasionally be due to other
viruses (parainfluenza, influenza, Coxsachie and Echo), or
bacteria (staphylococcus, streptococcus). Cerebrospinal fluid
changes are relatively common, and the meningoencephalitis
may be complicated by deafness.

6.6   **A C E**
The Monospot test is a simple and convenient method for
detecting the heterophil antibody, a marker of infectious
mononucleosis. Its limitations are that it is often negative inspite
of seroconversion in young children, and there are several
causes of false positive results, e.g. cytomegalovirus, leukaemia.
The virus infects B-lymphocytes and causes transient
impairment of cellular and humoral immunity. Fortunately, this is
almost always self-limiting and benign, but can be life
threatening if the immune system is already defective.

6.7   **B E**
Pertussis is not uncommon in young infants, particularly if they
are in contact with older non-immunized family members.
Infants typically present with apnoeic attacks or a diffuse
bronchopneumonia. Exact confirmation depends on growth of
Bordetella pertussis on fresh blood media (Bordet-Gengou agar).
A marked lymphocytosis is very suggestive. Erythromycin
therapy eradicates the organism but is unlikely to shorten the
clinical course. The convalescent phase may be very prolonged
and marked by recurrent bouts of cough and vomiting.

6.8   **B C**
The great majority of infection at all ages is by the respiratory
route. Populations drinking raw milk may develop cervical
lymph node or gut involvement.
    Young children are less able to contain primary tuberculosis
infection, and are especially vulnerable to systemic spread,
miliary tuberculosis, and meningitis. While older children may
show the characteristic features of TB, namely fever, night
sweats, weight loss, cough and haemoptysis, younger children
often have less specific symptoms. They are more likely to
present with irritability, high fever and toxicity. The tuberculin
response may not convert to positive for 2–3 months and may
be no help when a correct diagnosis is urgently required.
    Young children are most unlikely to have cavitating lung
disease and infectious sputum. When critically ill, they require all
the facilities of a comprehensively equipped paediatric unit.

6.9   Kawasaki disease

   A   causes conjunctivitis
   B   is caused by rickettsial infection
   C   produces thrombocytopenia
   D   produces coronary artery disease
   E   is an indication for intravenous gamma globulin therapy

6.10   The following classification of vaccines is correct

   A   tuberculosis (BCG) is a killed bacterial vaccine
   B   pertussis is a toxoid
   C   measles is a live viral vaccine
   D   rubella is a killed viral vaccine
   E   diphtheria is a killed bacterial vaccine

6.11   Live vaccines are contraindicated in

   A   children receiving replacement corticosteroid therapy
   B   children receiving immunosuppressive treatment
   C   children with cystic fibrosis
   D   children with severe eczema
   E   before age 3 months in infants born at gestation below 30
         weeks

(Answers overleaf)

6.9   **A D E**
Kawasaki disease is diagnosed on clinical criteria; prolonged
fever, conjunctivitis, pharyngitis, variable rash, cervical
lymphadenopathy, high ESR and thrombocytosis. The
aetiological agent has so far eluded definition, although it may
be the result of a toxin acting as a superantigen and triggering
widespread immune activation. Recognition is important so that
measures can be taken to reduce the mortality and morbidity
associated with myocarditis and coronary artery aneurysms.
Kawasaki disease is now one of the most common causes of
acquired heart disease in the young. Multicentre studies have
shown that prompt high dosage regimens of intravenous
gamma globulin reduce coronary heart disease. This disease
also provides one of the few indications for aspirin therapy in
children.

6.10 **C**
BCG (Bacillus Calmette-Guerin) is a freeze-dried attenuated
bovine strain. Pertussis vaccine is derived from killed organisms
of several serotypes of Bordetella pertussis. Current research is
directed towards identifying and synthesizing safer and more
effective constituents of the organisms. Rubella vaccine is a
freeze-dried suspension of live attenuated virus grown in tissue
culture. Diptheria vaccine is a formol inactivated toxoid
adsorbed to a mineral carrier.

6.11 **B**
No child should be denied immunization without considering the
potential penalties for both individual and society. Impaired
immunity provides the main contraindication to the use of live
vaccines; e.g. congenital immune deficiency or patients
receiving immunosuppressive therapy or high-dose
corticosteroids. Special risk groups such as those with asthma
or congenital heart disease should be immunized as a matter of
priority. Premature infants should be immunized according to
the recommended schedule commencing 2 months from birth.
   Immunization against Infectious Disease (HMSO 1992)
provides valuable guidance, particularly on problem cases
including children with HIV.

6.12 Meningococcal infection

   A is more frequent after age 10 years
   B is more frequent during outbreaks of influenza-like illness
   C is an indication for immediate parenteral therapy
   D is an indication for oral penicillin prophylaxis to family contacts
   E can be prevented using a polyvalent vaccine

6.13 Toxocara canis (dog roundworm)

   A is a recognized cause of blindness
   B is a recognized cause of epilepsy
   C may be eradicated with antihelminthics
   D is present in the majority of puppies
   E causes fever, cough and bronchospasm

(Answers overleaf)

6.12 **B C**
The age group between 3 months and 1 year is most affected by
meningococcal disease. A survey in Wales showed an attack
rate of 83 per 100 000 in infants aged under 1 year compared
with 1 per 100 000 in adults. There is a lesser peak in
adolescents.

The majority of victims are previously healthy and infection is
acquired by contact with a carrier. Carriage and spread appear
to increase in a temporal relationship with community outbreaks
of viral influenza-like illness.

Parenteral penicillin remains the drug of choice and must be
administered as soon as there is a clinical suspicion of the
disease. A number of countries including the UK have
encountered bacterial isolates with a reduced susceptibility to
penicillin but resistance is not yet a management problem.
Rifampicin is the currently recommended drug to eradicate
meningococcus in household contacts and in others who may
have had mouth-to-mouth or saliva contact. Household contacts
are 140 times more likely to be infected than the general
population.

Group B meningococci account for about 60% of cases in the
UK but capsular components have proved poorly immunogenic,
and no effective safe vaccine is currently available.
Polysaccharide vaccines against groups A and C are available
and are licensed for use in travellers to countries where these
strains are endemic.

6.13 **A B D E**
Puppies and lactating bitches shed huge quantities of Toxocara
canis eggs into the environment, and soil sampling shows
widespread contamination in parks and play areas frequented by
dogs. The eggs have thick shells and may survive for years until
ingested. The larvae then penetrate the gut wall and migrate
through the tissues, especially to liver, lungs, muscle and brain.
In the human, three main clinical syndromes are recognized:
visceral larva migrans (fever, malaise, bronchospasm, poor
weight gain with hepatosplenomegaly and lymphadenopathy),
ocular larva migrans, and covert toxocariasis. A single larva may
cause unilateral blindness.

The value of antihelminthics has not been proven and therapy
is primarily symptomatic. Prevention is a formidable public
health exercise aimed at reducing dog infestation and dog
access to children's areas.

6.14   The following have a recognized association

  A   Roseola infantum (exanthem subitum) and febrile
      convulsions
  B   parvovirus B19 and Erythema infectiosum (slapped face
      disease)
  C   varicella and cerebellar ataxia
  D   cytomegalovirus and sensorineural deafness
  E   Herpes simplex and chronic fatigue syndrome

(Answer overleaf)

6.14 **A B C D**
Roseola infantum is a common if infrequently diagnosed
infection of young children resulting in mild upper respiratory
tract symptoms and a high fever which may precipitate febrile
convulsions. The presumed viral pathogen remained elusive
until the isolation of human Herpes virus-6 which is tropic for
T-lymphocytes.

Human parvovirus B19, a small DNA virus, is also relatively
common and potentially important not only as a cause of a
childhood rash but also because infection may be complicated
by arthritis, neuritis, meningitis and transient marrow
hypoplasia. The latter is a trigger of aplastic crises in children
with haemoglobinopathies. Parvovirus has also been linked to
fetal loss and non-immune hydrops.

7. Hazards

7.1 **Accidental injury in children under age 5 years**
- A occurs predominantly in the home
- B is more likely when there is only one child in the household
- C is more frequent in single parent families
- D is less likely when there has been previous accidental injury
- E should be brought to the attention of the family's Health Visitor

7.2 **A child with a history of head injury must be admitted to hospital**
- A if he momentarily lost consciousness
- B if there is a fine fracture of a temporal bone
- C if there is superficial bruising over the mastoid area
- D if there is bleeding from the ear
- E if there is a conjunctival haemorrhage without definable limit

7.3 **Cerebral oedema**
- A is less common after head injury in children than in adults
- B is aggravated by retention of CO_2
- C is suggested by falling blood pressure
- D is suggested by bradycardia
- E is suggested by pulsus paradoxus

7.4 **A child admitted following paraffin (kerosene oil) ingestion**
- A should be given an emetic
- B should have a gastric lavage
- C is liable to develop pneumonitis
- D is likely to develop severe diarrhoea
- E should be fasted for 24 hours

(Answers overleaf)

7.1   A C E

It is entirely appropriate that accident reduction should be one of the targets of *The Health of the Nation*. The death rate for children aged under 15 years in the UK was 6.7 per 100 000 population in 1990, and the target for 2005 is a reduction of 33%. Most accidents in under 5s occur in the home and are preventable. Sadly surveys in Nottingham showed a progressive rise between 1987 and 1991, and identified risk factors included: more than three children in the family, young maternal age, single parent families, deprivation, previous accidental injury and family stress. There was a lack of awareness of the importance of safety equipment, e.g. stairgates, fireguards and safety catches on doors and windows. Health Visitors are well placed to promote safety in the home and facilitate equipment 'loan schemes' for families on low income.

7.2   A B D E

Admission criteria will vary from hospital to hospital; most would admit for observation any child with complicating signs or symptoms. Simple fine skull fractures are usually innocent but beware of those in the territory of the middle meningeal artery.

7.3   B D

The soft child's skull increases the risk of brain distortion and oedema. Hypoventilation and hypercapnia aggravate the oedema. A falling pulse and a rising blood pressure suggest increased intracranial pressure.

7.4   C

Aspiration and pneumonitis are the main hazards and therefore emesis and gastric lavage are contraindicated. Diarrhoea is uncommon and a high milk intake is beneficial.

7.5   **The following are recommended treatments for poisoning**
  A   oral ipecauanah for alkaline ingestion
  B   intravenous N-acetylcysteine for paracetamol poisoning
  C   chlorpromazine for dystonic reactions
  D   oral bicarbonate for acid ingestion
  E   intravenous methylene blue for nitrate-induced
       methaemoglobinaemia

7.6   **Lead poisoning may present with**
  A   convulsions
  B   renal colic
  C   abdominal pain
  D   weariness and irritability
  E   swollen joints

7.7   **Severe head injuries**
  A   are responsible for at least 20% of deaths in the 5–15 age
       group
  B   occur most commonly in children who are car passengers
  C   occur predominantly within 2 km of the child's home
  D   are equally common in all social classes
  E   are more common in boys

(Answers overleaf)

7.5   **B E**
Vomiting must not be induced in either acid or alkaline
ingestion. There is no value to attempts at pH neutralization.
Apart from rinsing the mouth to remove residual alkaline, the
child should be kept nil by mouth until specialist evaluation,
possibly including endoscopy, has been performed. Ingested
acids may be diluted by drinking milk and water.
     Phenothiazines have a very limited role in paediatric practice,
not least because of the risk of dystonic reactions.

7.6   **A C D**
Lead poisoning is becoming an increasingly rare event due to
the limits imposed on the use of lead in paint manufacture and
the disappearance of lead water pipes and tanks. It can be
difficult to recognize, causing anything from vague abdominal
pain and weariness to convulsions.

7.7   **A C E**
One in 20 children per year has a head injury. Fortunately, the
vast majority are mild but 25% of deaths in the age group 5–15
years are caused by severe head injury, and 20–30% of
survivors of severe injury have motor and learning difficulties.
     Pedestrians and those engaged in unsafe play are most at risk.
The accidents commonly happen near home and in the early
evening. Boys and especially those from deprived backgrounds
are particularly at risk.

8. Airways and lungs

8.1 The following are recognized causes of pharyngitis
A influenza virus
B Epstein-Barr virus
C corynebacterium species
D *Streptococcus pyogenes*
E *Mycoplasma pneumoniae*

8.2 Acute laryngotracheo bronchitis (croup)
A is usually caused by viral infection
B is usually preceded by other upper respiratory symptoms
C of sufficient severity to merit hospital admission is best treated in a mist tent with added oxygen
D associated with restlessness is an indication for sedation
E is not benefited by corticosteroid therapy

8.3 Tonsillectomy is indicated for
A persistent cervical lymphadenopathy
B speech distortion
C cor pulmonale due to upper airway obstruction
D disruption of schooling due to repeated sore throats
E asymptomatic asymmetrical tonsillar enlargement

8.4 Persistent stridor is caused by
A vocal cord paralysis
B congenital hypothyroidism
C laryngomalacia
D tracheal haemangioma
E vitamin D deficiency

(Answers overleaf)

8.1   **A B C D E**
The majority of infectious pharyngitis is viral in origin. The
possibility of group A β-haemolytic streptococcus
(Streptococcus pyogenes) infection continues to influence
prescribing habits in spite of the current rarity of rheumatic fever
in the developed world. Early antibacterial therapy in
streptococcal pharyngitis does shorten the illness, prevent
suppurative complications, and lessens family and school
disruption. The difficulty is confidently diagnosing streptococcal
pharyngitis without recourse to laboratory facilities.

8.2   **A B E**
Influenza, para-influenza and respiratory syncytial virus account
for most cases. Coryza is a frequent antecedent. An abrupt
onset in a previously well child raises the possibility of acute
epiglottitis or an inhaled foreign body.
    Steam inhalation, as provided in the bathroom, is a useful
measure in the home. It is unlikely that the child, frightened by
admission to hospital, benefits from being confined within a
mist tent. Nursing observations certainly suffer. Added oxygen
does nothing to relieve the airway problem and may delay
recognition of impending obstruction. Restlessness is an
important sign of hypoxaemia and sedatives should be avoided.
The child will sleep peacefully when his airway permits.

8.3   **C D**
The indications for tonsillectomy are as difficult to define as they
are to justify. They are likely to differ depending on whether you
consult a paediatrician or an ENT surgeon. Persistent tonsillar
enlargement is not an indication unless it causes symptoms.
Children often have asymmetrical tonsils. Chronic upper airways
obstruction may be manifest by snoring, disturbed sleep,
daytime tiredness and failure to thrive. A few such children have
chronic hypoventilation of such severity that it causes
pulmonary hypertension and right heart failure.

8.4   **A C D**
There are many causes of stridor. They are most readily
subdivided into causes within the lumen, in the wall of the
airway, and structures outside compressing the airway.
Laryngeal nerve paralysis may be bilateral or unilateral. It may
be an isolated finding or secondary to other structural or
neurological disorders. Laryngomalacia is usually a benign
condition and is the label often attached to infants whose
symptoms do not call for formal evaluation such as endoscopy.

8.5 Acute bronchiolitis
- A is caused by a single strain of respiratory synctial virus
- B is readily transmitted by nursing staff
- C is an indication for short-term prednisolone
- D is a cause of hepatomegaly
- E can be prevented by active immunization

8.6 Community-acquired pneumonia in childhood has a recognized association with
- A klebsiella sp.
- B respiratory synctial virus (RSV)
- C *Streptococcus pneumoniae*
- D *Streptococcus pyogenes*
- E *Mycoplasma pneumoniae*

8.7 Characteristic features of pneumococcal pneumonia include
- A meningism
- B delirium
- C a petechial rash
- D hypochondrial pain
- E arthritis

8.8 *Mycoplasma pneumoniae* infection
- A typically produces a pneumonia with widespread crepitations (rales)
- B is suggested by the production of IgM antibody capable of agglutinating red cells
- C is a recognized cause of arthritis
- D is a recognized cause of erythema multiforme
- E is responsive to amoxicillin

(Answers overleaf)

8.5   **B**
Molecular epidemiology has established that multiple subgroups circulate during epidemics. Analysis of viral strains reveals patterns of cross-infection within units. Most nosocomial outbreaks originate from multiple sources and it is important to take measures to reduce spread, especially to the very young and the vulnerable such as those with lung or cardiac disease. Effective measures include cohort nursing and scrupulous hand washing.

Management is primarily directed at supportive nursing with attention to oxygenation and feeding. There is controversy as the value of inhaled bronchodilator therapy and there is little evidence to justify corticosteroids. Ribavirin, a specific antiviral agent, has made little impact on disease severity.

Acute bronchiolitis produces lung air trapping and depression of the diaphragm so that the liver is more readily palpable, but not enlarged.

Bioengineering is being exploited in an attempt to design recombinant RSV vaccines but we are still some distance from safe and effective preparations.

8.6   **B C E**
Pneumonia remains an important cause of childhood death in developing countries, and is a leading cause of primary care consultation and hospitalization in Western countries. Despite modern microbiological techniques the differentiation between viral and bacterial pathogens remains a problem. In a recent study of hospitalized children, 20% were defined as having a viral pathogen (RSV will be conspicuous during epidemics), 15% had a bacterial cause, and another 15% had mixed viral/bacterial aetiology. *Mycoplasma pneumoniae* needs to be considered when initial treatment with penicillin fails, although it is uncertain whether erythromycin shortens the illness duration.

8.7   **A B D**
Children with pneumococcal pneumonia may present to the surgeon with abdominal pain, or have a lumbar puncture for suspected meningitis before they have chest X-rays which demonstrate the diagnosis. The abrupt high fever may cause delirium.

8.8   **B C D**
Mycoplasma pneumonia is one of the commonest respiratory tract pathogens. However, the majority of infected individuals do not seek medical intervention; less than 10% have clinically apparent pneumonia. Those who do present with persistent cough sometimes have minimal chest signs but conspicuously abnormal chest X-rays.

Mycoplasma infection can produce a wide range of systemic complications including hepatitis, nephritis, arthritis, meningo-encephalitis, peripheral neuropathy and mucocutaneous reactions.

Recommended therapy is a 2-week course of either erythromycin or tetracycline.

8.9   Epiglottitis
  A   is not usually associated with a high fever
  B   is associated with *Haemophilus influenza* bacteraemia
  C   produces a characteristic barking cough
  D   is confirmed by depressing the tongue and observing the characteristic supraglottic oedema
  E   necessitates elective endotracheal intubation

8.10   Recognized features of asthma include
  A   nocturnal cough
  B   apnoeic attacks
  C   exercise-induced wheeze
  D   pectus excavatum (funnel chest)
  E   Kussmaul breathing

8.11   Asthma
  A   has a prevalence of between 2 and 10 per 1000 in UK schoolchildren
  B   is more prevalent in boys
  C   is more prevalent in older children
  D   is more strongly associated with house dust mite than any other identified allergen
  E   is commonly overtreated

8.12   The following drug side-effects are recognized
  A β_2-agonists and interference with hand-writing
  B   theophylline and behaviour disorder
  C   inhaled corticosteroids and angioneurotic oedema
  D   inhaled cromoglycate and cough
  E   inhaled ipratropium (Atrovent) and excess salivation

(Answers overleaf)

8.9   **B E**
Epiglottitis must be considered in a child with rapid onset of
fever, toxicity, difficulty in swallowing and phonation, and with
evolving signs of upper airway obstruction. It results in a
muffled voice with inability of cough. No attempt should be
made to examine the pharynx other than as part of endotracheal
intubation. Until this is possible the child should be kept as calm
as possible and in an upright position.

8.10   **A C**
Asthma may coexist with a chest deformity such as pectus
excavatum, but is usually associated with chronic hyperinflation
and a barrel-shaped chest. Kussmaul breathing is a term
reserved for the deep breathing pattern secondary to metabolic
acidosis.

8.11   **B D**
Surveys of asthma prevalence reveal figures of between 2 and
15% with increasing support for the higher end of this range.
The male:female ratio is consistently reported as being
approximately 2:1 but there is no agreed explanation for this sex
difference. Asthma is more prevalent in younger children, first
coming to attention in the preschool years and abating during
puberty. In spite of the increasing awareness of asthma
symptoms in young children, delayed recognition and
inadequate attention to therapy continue to handicap large
numbers of children. Excessive bronchodilator therapy has been
suggested as a contributory factor in the still unacceptable level
of asthma mortality, but undertreatment of deteriorating
bronchospasm is a far greater problem.

8.12   **A B D**
Side-effects have been reported for all types of therapy used in
asthma. It is important to be alert to these as they may
contribute to poor compliance.
   β_2-adrenoceptor stimulants may cause hand tremor,
tachycardia, and sleep disturbance. The hand tremor can
interfere with school work and the child may be labelled as
clumsy.
   Theophylline has in the past been used at relatively high
dosage with the risk of side-effects including headaches,
insomnia and reduced cognitive function.
   Inhaled corticosteroids at appropriate dosage are relatively
free of side-effects apart from hoarseness and oral candidiasis.
Rinsing the mouth after dosage is advised. Powder inhalers in
which the active drug is associated with a lactose carrier may
provoke cough and transient bronchospasm.
   Ipratropium is an antimuscarinic bronchodilator and may
produce a dry mouth.

8.13 Recognized presenting features of cystic fibrosis include
  A neonatal small bowel obstruction
  B perioral and perianal skin rash
  C rectal prolapse
  D bronchiectasis
  E persistent stridor

8.14 Standard management of cystic fibrosis includes
  A severely restricted fat intake
  B pancreatic enzyme supplementation
  C multivitamin supplementation
  D residential schooling
  E organizing exemption from physical education

8.15 Otitis media with effusion (glue ear)
  A has a peak incidence at about age 2 years
  B is limited to children who have a history of acute otitis media
  C is more frequent in children with high arched palates
  D is more frequent in children exposed to passive cigarette smoking
  E is a progressive disorder unless interrupted by grommet (ventilator tube) insertion

(Answers overleaf)

8.13 **A C D**
Small bowel obstruction due to inspissated viscid meconium is
the presenting problem in 10–15% of children with cystic
fibrosis. Rectal prolapse in a malnourished toddler should alert
you to the possibility of cystic fibrosis. Chronic diarrhoea in a
weaning infant who also has refractory dermatitis of mouth,
anus and digits raises the possibility of acrodermatitis
enteropathica. This is a rare and potentially fatal disorder
associated with defective zinc absorption.

8.14 **B C**
It is important to emphasize a good caloric intake without
restricting fat other than to avoid abdominal pain and offensive
flatus. Tailoring pancreatic enzyme replacement is the more
important contribution. Children should be encouraged to attend
normal schools and to participate in the full educational
curriculum, including as much physical exercie as they can cope
with.

8.15 **A C D**
Otitis media with effusion (chronic secretory otitis media, glue
ear) is primarily a disorder of young children with a peak
incidence at around 2 years and a smaller peak at school entry.
Infection is an important aetiological factor but not all children
have a history of acute otitis media. Atopy and craniofacial
abnormalities, which interfere with Eustachian tube function, are
other factors. Breastfeeding has been reported as being
protective and cigarette smoke exposure as contributory.
   Otitis media with effusion shows a tendency to spontaneous
resolution but it may interfere with hearing, language
development and behaviour in young children. The topic which
continues to challenge ENT surgeons and health planners is
whether surgery is justified in the many children presenting with
glue ears and conductive deafness. Grommet insertion is the
commonest childhood surgical procedure in the UK. Middle ear
ventilation does produce an immediate improvement in hearing
and is probably important to children with severe conductive
deafness. It is less certain that language development is
improved. Grommets fall out or become obstructed in 9–10
months, and the procedure can produce tympanic membrane
scarring and other morbidity.

9. Heart

9.1 **The following signs are helpful in the recognition of heart failure in infancy**
  A a resting heart rate greater than 180 per minute
  B an elevated jugular venous pulse
  C hepatomegaly
  D a loud first heart sound
  E sweating

9.2 **The following may be present in a child with a normal heart**
  A a continuous murmur
  B a thrill
  C an isolated diastolic murmur
  D a third heart sound
  E ventricular extrasystoles

9.3 **In children with atrial septal (ostium secundum) defects**
  A symptoms do not usually develop until adult life
  B the associated systolic murmur is created by turbulent flow across the atrial septal defect
  C delayed closure of the pulmonary valve produces 'fixed splitting' of the second heart sound
  D a right bundle branch block is a common ECG finding
  E there is a significant risk of infective endocarditis

9.4 **Ventricular septal defects**
  A usually occur in the muscular part of the septum
  B close spontaneously in more than 50% of affected children
  C have a benign outcome if accompanied by accentuation of the second heart sound
  D causing a large left to right shunt result in the presence of a mid-diastolic murmur
  E result in a significant risk of infective endocarditis

(Answers overleaf)

9.1   **A C E**
The average resting pulse rate in the first year is approximately 120 per minute, with the upper limit at 160–170. The short neck of infancy denies exploitation of the jugular venous pulse, but the liver rapidly reflects congestive cardiac failure. Myocarditis and cardiac failure result in poorer quality heart sounds. A low grade fever and sweating are important features of heart failure in infancy.

9.2   **A D E**
An innocent venous hum produces a blowing continuous murmur above and below the clavicles. It may be abolished by rotating the neck or compressing the internal jugular vein. Other innocent murmurs are ejection or mid-systolic. Neither a thrill nor a diastolic murmur are compatible with this diagnosis. Both the third heart sound and ventricular extrasystoles may occur in healthy children.

9.3   **A C D**
The ejection systolic murmur is caused by excessive blood flow through the normal pulmonary valve. There is no murmur directly related to the defect.
  Right bundle branch block is present in 95% of ostium secundum defects.
  Infective endocarditis is a negligible risk in this disorder.

9.4   **B D E**
The defect usually lies in the membranous part of the septum, immediately below the aortic valve.
  Spontaneous closure is common and usually occurs during the first year of life, although it can occur later.
  A disappearing murmur accompanied by a loud palpable second heart sound indicates the evolution of pulmonary hypertension and cessation of the left to right shunt. Eventually reversal of the shunt results in cyanosis. This result is described as the Eisenmenger complex.

9.5 Patent ductus arteriosus
- A occurs more commonly in babies born prematurely
- B results in central cyanosis
- C produces a systolic murmur which may or may not continue into diastole
- D is seldom associated with a palpable thrill
- E carries a significant risk of bacterial endocarditis

9.6 In children with Fallot tetralogy
- A central cyanosis is a consistent feature during infancy
- B heart failure is a rare complication
- C episodic loss of consciousness is a recognized feature
- D the murmur of a ventricular septal defect is usually present
- E the lung fields are polycythaemic

9.7 Transposition of the great arteries
- A usually results in early progressive cyanosis
- B is not usually accompanied by a heart murmur
- C produces central cyanosis which improves in 100% oxygen
- D produces plethoric lung fields
- E is an indication for atrial septostomy

9.8 Coarctation of the aorta
- A is usually proximal to the left subclavian artery
- B results in an ejection systolic murmur audible in the interscapular area
- C is seldom symptomatic in school age children
- D is an isolated disorder in approximately 90% of cases
- E results in biventricular hypertrophy

9.9 Supraventricular tachycardia
- A is characterized by an abnormally fast and irregular pulse rate
- B is associated with a structurally normal heart in the majority of affected children
- C gradually slows in response to carotid sinus pressure
- D is associated with the Wolff–Parkinson–White syndrome
- E having its onset in infancy is usually associated with a good prognosis

(Answers overleaf)

9.5   **A C E**
Patent ductus arteriosus is a common problem in immature
infants, frequently delaying recovery from respiratory distress
syndrome. Fortunately, closure may be promoted by medical
means such as careful fluid management and the administration
of a prostaglandin synthetase inhibitor, indomethacin. The
classical murmur is continuous and accompanied by a thrill. It is,
however, commonly limited to systole in low birthweight
infants. Bacterial endocarditis is a potential hazard even when
the ductus is very narrow and unlikely to cause heart failure.

9.6   **B C**
Except in the most severe cases of pulmonary artery stenosis,
cyanosis develops later in infancy. The cyanosis may only be
apparent after crying or other exertion. The transient
interruptions of pulmonary blood flow can acutely impair
cerebral oxygenation and result in loss of consciousness. The
systolic murmur originates from the pulmonary outflow and not
the septal defect, the ventricular pressures being similar.

9.7   **A B D E**
Central cyanosis develops early as closure of the foramen ovale
and ductus causes isolation of the pulmonary and systemic
circulations. Cyanotic congenital heart disease fails to respond
to the administration of even 100% oxygen.

9.8   **B C**
Coarctation is usually close to the site of the ductus and just
distal to the origin of the left subclavian artery. Severe, complex
cases present as heart failure in infancy but most affected
children are asymptomatic. Ideally they are diagnosed following
routine examination. Associated disorders occur in up to 50%
and include other heart lesions and aneurysms of the cerebral
arteries.

9.9   **B D E**
Supraventricular tachycardia produces a fast, regular pulse rate
which does not gradually slow in response to carotid sinus
pressure. The majority of affected infants have structurally
normal hearts and have a good prognosis for resolution of the
problem as long as their initial episodes are recognized and
treated appropriately. Older children and those with persisting
attacks are more likely to have significant heart disease, e.g.
Ebstein anomaly or corrected transposition.

9.10 Heart failure in infancy

A   presents with poor feeding
B   forehead sweating
C   is most commonly due to a large right to left shunt
D   is delayed while pulmonary vascular resistance remains high
E   may improve spontaneously because of a secondary
     increase in pulmonary vascular resistance

9.11 Blood pressure

A   increases in relation to height
B   should be measured routinely in all pre-school children
C   is artificially decreased by using too narrow an arm cuff
D   elevation is associated with neuroblastoma
E   elevation is associated with heamolytic–uraemic syndrome

(Answers overleaf)

9.10   **A B D E**

Congenital heart disease may first manifest as acute circulatory collapse in early infancy, in which situation a left-sided obstructive pathology is probable, or as heart failure usually secondary to a large left to right shunt. The time-scale of onset of heart failure is determined by the balance between shunt size and pulmonary vascular resistance. The normally rapid fall in pulmonary bed resistance may be delayed until 4–8 weeks at which age shunt volume becomes sufficient to precipitate failure. In a minority of infants pulmonary resistance remains high or rises secondary to the increased flow. If undetected this pulmonary hypertension may evolve to the Eisenmenger syndrome.

9.11   **A D E**

Published standards relate blood pressure to gender and age or height, and show centile distribution for systolic and diastolic values.

Practical difficulties and the infrequency of hypertension in healthy young children make routine screening an unrewarding exercise. Health workers should, however, measure blood pressure in children where symptoms might possibly reflect renal, neurological, cardiac or endocrine disease. A family history of hypertension is also an indication.

It is a common error to use too narrow an arm cuff. The cuff should fit around at least two-thirds of the length of the upper arm.

10. Gut

10.1 Mesenteric adenitis, rather than acute appendicitis, is suggested by

A a high fever, temperature above 38°C
B variably situated abdominal pain
C periumbilical tenderness
D pharyngitis
E ketonuria

10.2 The following may be presenting features of acute appendicitis

A acute constipation
B diarrhoea lasting more than 24 hours
C pyuria, 20–50 white blood cells/mm³
D left-sided abdominal pain
E a limp

10.3 The following features increase the likelihood of an organic basis for recurrent abdominal pain

A pain awaking the child at night
B periumbilical pain
C loin pain
D bile-stained vomiting
E associated headache

10.4 Intussusception is suggested by

A the gradual onset of abdominal pain
B associated vomiting
C the early association of fever
D calm appearance of the infant between episodes of pain
E constipation

(Answers overleaf)

10.1 **A B D**
Varying abdominal pain in association with systemic features such as an upper respiratory tract infection or generalized lymphadenopathy favour mesenteric adenitis but there are few hard and fast rules. The cautious clinician relies on serial observations to establish minimal abdominal tenderness in two or more areas which often change, failure of progression and resolution.

10.2 **A B C D E**
All children with acute persistent abdominal pain should be assessed in case of acute appendicitis but there is an extensive differential diagnosis. The clinical diagnosis usually hinges on demonstrating objective signs of local or general peritonitis, localized tenderness and guarding. In young children guarding may be difficult to elicit reliably, and in the very young fever, irritability and immobility may be main clues to peritonitis. An appendix and its associated abscess may be separated from the abdominal wall by other inflamed organs leading to a range of potentially misleading signs.

10.3 **A C D**
Recurrent abdominal pain is one of the commonest problems encountered in paediatrics. In most cases a manifestly healthy child presents with several brief episodes of central abdominal colicy pain, and abdominal examination is normal. Surgical problems usually produce more severe and prolonged pain. Pain which awakes a child from sleep, or which is localized away from the periumbilical area, is more likely to be organic. Bile-stained vomiting is an important sign and raises the possibility of malrotation and volvulus. All too frequently prodromal episodes of partial obstruction are overlooked and the child subsequently presents with infarcted gut.

10.4 **B D**
Awake or asleep the infant with intussusception suddenly cries out in agony, and the mother can often recall the exact time of onset. Reflex vomiting is a common symptom, as is diarrhoea. Fever is usually a late and hopefully avoidable consequence of peritonitis. Between the attacks of pain children are described as calm and preoccupied. Presented with such a characteristic history nobody should overlook this diagnosis.

10.5 Oral rehydration solutions used to treat mild-to-moderate diarrhoea
  A contain glucose in order to prevent hypoglycaemia
  B contain glucose to facilitate absorption of water and electrolytes
  C contain sodium 100–150 mmol/l
  D contain potassium 100–150 mmol/l
  E contain an alkalizing agent

10.6 Enterotoxins are important in the pathogenesis of gastroenteritis due to
  A *Escherichia coli*
  B *Giardia lamblia*
  C *Staphylococcus aureus*
  D salmonella species
  E *Vibrio cholerae*

10.7 Giardiasis
  A is uncommon in industrialized societies
  B is spread by the waterborne route
  C is spread by person-to-person contact
  D causes chronic malabsorption
  E is controlled by the use of piperazine

10.8 The following measures are appropriate to the management of a 4-month-old infant with an 18-hour history of vomiting and diarrhoea
  A the prescription of a glucose electrolyte preparation for 48 hours
  B the prescription of oral metoclopramide to reduce vomiting
  C the prescription of oral diphenoxylate hydrochloride (Lomotil) to reduce diarrhoea
  D the cessation of milk formula feeds until the return of normally formed bowel actions
  E broad-spectrum antibacterial therapy

(Answers overleaf)

10.5 **B E**
Oral rehydration therapy is one of the most important and cost-effective tools in the world paediatric formulary. Glucose or a readily digestable source of glucose polymer enhances intestinal absorption of sodium and water. The energy content is, however, insufficient to sustain metabolism; an adequate source of nutrition should be reintroduced as soon as possible despite persistence of diarrhoea. Oral rehydration solutions marketed in areas where gastroenteritis and dehydration are less severe contain sodium in the range 30–75 mmol/l. WHO promotes a stronger solution, sodium 90 mmol/l, to cater for more severe electrolyte loss and it also recommends additional sources of water or continuation of breastfeeding.

10.6 **A C E**
Enterotoxigenic *E. coli* and *Vibrio cholerae* attach to the small intestinal brush border via surface proteins (adhesins) and release protein exotoxins which stimulate fluid and electrolyte excretion. The enterotoxins produced by shigella, campylobacter and yersinia are still being researched. Non-typhoid salmonella is regarded as being predominantly invasive resulting in degeneration and vacuolation of the brush border.

10.7 **B C D**
Giardiasis is a worldwide infection affecting children and adults. It is prevalent in day nurseries catering for children in nappies. Spread is both by personal contact and by contaminated water supplies. The majority of older patients are either asymptomatic or demonstrate diarrhoea and abdominal discomfort. Patients under age 5 years and those who are immunocompromized are more prone to heavy infestation with mucosal inflammation, and resulting anorexia, malabsorption and growth impairment. Metronidazole is the recommended therapy but eradication may be difficult in the face of repeated exposure or defective immunity.

10.8 **A**
Glucose electrolyte preparations either manufactured by pharmaceutical companies or created from ingredients within the community are usually sufficient to treat gastroenteritis. Young dehydrated infants are particularly vulnerable to the side-effects of metoclopramide and diphenoxylate, and neither is justified. Infants, expecially those already threatened by malnutrition, must not be deprived of milk for any longer than necessary. As a general rule, frequent small volume milk feeds can be reintroduced as soon as vomiting has ceased and dehydration has been largely corrected. Antibacterial therapy plays little part in the management of infective gastroenteritis unless it is established that an at-risk infant is infected by a potentially invasive organism.

10.9 Coeliac disease
    A   normally results in villous and crypt atrophy within the small
        intestinal mucosa
    B   is most unlikely in a child presenting with poor weight gain
        and constipation
    C   results in hypoproteinaemia
    D   requires elimination of wheat and rye from the diet
    E   is caused by permanent intolerance to glutein

10.10 Constipation
    A   may be defined as pain on defaecation
    B   may be defined as delay in defaecation
    C   may be defined as difficulty in defaecation
    D   in early infancy is frequently due to lack of dietary fibre
    E   with temporary improvement after rectal examination is
        consistent with Hirschsprung disease

10.11 Hirschsprung disease
    A   is more frequent in premature infants
    B   results from absence of ganglion cells in the myenteric and
        submucosal nerve plexuses
    C   is a cause of persistent faecal soiling
    D   produces diarrhoea and circulatory collapse in early infancy
    E   is associated with passive dilatation of the aganglionic bowel

(Answers overleaf)

10.9   **C D E**
The relative contribution of immunological and biochemical mechanisms provoked by exposure to the gliadin component of glutein has not been resolved, but it is accepted that biopsy proven coeliac disease is a permanent disorder. The typical biopsy shows villous damage with crypt hyperplasia.

Although the majority of children present with diarrhoea, anorexia may reduce food intake to such an extent that constipation becomes conspicuous. Hypoproteinaemia is a feature of malabsorption and may be so severe as to result in oedema.

10.10 **A B C E**
The infrequent passage of hard or excessively bulky stools is a valid cause for complaint. Long intervals between stools may be innocent if the stools are soft; this may be the case in breastfed infants.

Most constipated infants have hard stools due to relative fluid lack and it is important to add milk-free drinks in later infancy. Lack of fibre becomes an issue if toddlers and young children remain too dependent on milk and a selection of low fibre solids. If constipation persists in an infant despite attention to fluid intake, then a structural cause needs to be considered. Milder degrees of anorectal stenosis may be temporally relieved by rectal examination or suppository insertion. Additional clues favouring Hirschsprung disease are a history of delayed passage of meconium, abdominal distension, failure to thrive, and episodes of diarrhoea interrupting constipation.

10.11 **B D**
Hirschsprung disease has an incidence of around 1 in 5000 births and, unlike most other congenital gut disorders, is not more frequent in premature infants. The aganglionic segment is passively contracted and the majority of cases are capable of early diagnosis if sufficient attention is payed to delayed passage of meconium. Delayed recognition increases the risk of life threatening enterocolitis in which collapse and diarrhoea are features.

10.12 In a jaundiced infant, conjugated hyperbilirubinaemia is suggested by

    A urine which tests positive for urobilinogen
    B pale stools
    C elevated hepatic transaminase levels
    D bile-stained vomiting
    E a prolonged prothrombin time

10.13 Breast milk jaundice

    A is the most frequent cause of prolonged jaundice in term infants
    B is accompanied by a modest elevation of hepatic transaminase levels
    C is not an indication for the cessation of breastfeeding
    D is associated with pale stools
    E is likely to affect successive infants fed by the same mother

10.14 Hepatitis A

    A commonly presents as a gastroenteritis-like illness
    B has low infectivity prior to the icteric phase of the illness
    C protection is available in the form of an inactivated virus vaccine
    D is not transmitted by blood transfusion
    E is not associated with chronic hepatitis

(Answers overleaf)

10.12 **B   C   E**
Some 90% of infants become jaundiced in the days after birth but this should resolve within the first 2 weeks and not recur. Persistent or recurrent jaundice is an important sign of potentially severe liver disease, e.g. biliary atresia and α1-antitrypsin deficiency. In the UK, a national campaign 'Yellow Alert' has been launched to increase public and health professional awareness of early liver disease. Key components in preliminary assessment are to inspect the stools to ensure that they contain yellow or green pigment, to check the urine for the presence of bilirubin (not urobilinogen) and to take a blood sample for the measurement of total and conjugated bilirubin and liver function. It should be emphasized that infants with liver disease may look superficially healthy with adequate weight gain and no hepatosplenomegaly.

10.13 **C   E**
True breast milk jaundice is a relatively uncommon occurrence. Jaundice accompanying breastfeeding is common and usually transient, reflecting physiological jaundice accentuated by delayed fluid and calorie intake. A small number of mothers have successive babies displaying prolonged, moderate unconjugated hyperbilirubinaemia. A number of mechanisms have been proposed based on steroid, fatty acid or enzyme constituents of breast milk. Breast milk jaundice is innocent and resolves without having to disrupt feeding.

10.14 **A   C   E**
Hepatitis A virus is an RNA virus, the structure and genome of which have now been defined. Infection is widespread in areas where water supplies and food hygiene are suspect, and the majority of children become immune without recognized hepatitis. The main source of infection is virus shed into the stool in the late incubation period before biochemical and/or clinical hepatitis.

Hepatitis A vaccine is available and is recommended for non-immune travellers from developed countries to high risk areas. It is reported to have a protective efficacy of 97%.

Hepatitis A is conventionally spread by the faeco-oral route but transmission from a blood donor with prodromal hepatitis A is possible.

Hepatitis A can result in considerable short-term disability and inconvenience but fulminant hepatic failure occurs in less than 0.5% of recognized cases. Chronic hepatitis does not occur and if suspected an alternative explanation such as underlying α-1-antitrypsin deficiency has to be excluded.

10.15 Reye syndrome
- A refers to the association of hepatitis and encephalitis
- B typically evolves after apparently mild viral illness
- C has been linked to aspirin administration
- D is usually accompanied by jaundice
- E is a recognized cause of cirrhosis

10.16 Wilson disease
- A in childhood presents most commonly with neurological symptoms
- B may be reliably excluded by the presence of a normal serum caeruloplasmin level
- C is a cause of haemolytic anaemia
- D results in renal tubular damage
- E is inherited as an autosomal recessive disorder

10.17 Hepatosplenomegaly is a recognized feature of
- A chronic aggressive hepatitis
- B thalassaemia
- C portal hypertension due to portal vein thrombosis
- D neonatal Herpes simplex infection
- E haemorrhagic disease of the newborn

10.18 Galactosaemia
- A has a delayed presentation in breastfed as compared to formula fed infants
- B is reliably excluded by testing the urine for reducing substances
- C usually presents with jaundice, vomiting and diarrhoea
- D results from the deficiency of an enzyme specifically located in liver tissue
- E results in the early evolution of cataracts

(Answers overleaf)

10.15 **B C**
Reye syndrome is an important, although relatively rare, cause of acute encephalopathy in which there is no inflammatory or demyelinating component. The cerebral oedema is associated with a systemic derangement of mitochondrial function, most conspicuous in the liver where it results in microvesicular fatty infiltration and disturbed function.

The association with prior aspirin usage has been suggested by epidemiological studies. It also links with our understanding of the mechanism whereby aspirin may aggravate the mitochondrial detoxification processes already compromised by relative carnitine deficiency.

10.16 **C D E**
Childhood Wilson disease usually presents as a liver disorder; chronic hepatitis, cirrhosis or acute liver failure. It is rarely symptomatic before the age of 6 years. Ten to 15% of affected children have a normal caeruloplasmin level and where the clinical indications are strong, a liver copper estimation must be performed.

10.17 **A B D**
The liver of healthy infants may be palpable in the midclavicular line up to 4 cm below the costal margin. As it becomes more of a thoracic rather than abdominal organ, percussion becomes more relevant for determining size. The tip of the spleen may be palpable in slim healthy young children. It commonly becomes transiently palpable during infections.

The differential diagnosis of hepatosplenomegaly makes a formidable list, but careful history and examination will usually reveal other features which focus attention on an appropriate shorter list.

10.18 **C E**
Galactosaemia is rare, 1 in 70 000 births in the UK, but its characteristic presentation and its prompt response to dietary management demands that you are familiar with it! Both breast milk and conventional cow's milk formulae contain lactose and therefore galactose. Deficient galactose-1-phosphate uridyl transferase results in the accumulation of galactose-1-phosphate which acts as a multiorgan tissue toxin. This enzyme is present in red blood cells and is the basis of the diagnostic test. Galactosuria may be present but urine screening is unreliable.

11. Urinary tract and testes

11.1 The kidneys of the newborn infant

  A have approximately 50% of the adult complement of glomeruli

  B have reduced blood flow compared to mature kidneys

  C have an increased glomerular filtration rate compared to the adult after correction for body surface area

  D are less able to excrete a salt load compared to the adult

  E are less able to concentrate urine compared to the adult

11.2 Renal agenesis is associated with

  A oligohydramnios

  B congenital heart disease

  C limb contractures

  D sensorineural deafness

  E pulmonary hypoplasia

11.3 Posterior urethral valves

  A can present throughout childhood

  B are frequently associated with other major congenital anomalies

  C are frequently diagnosed in the antenatal period

  D may be excluded from diagnostic consideration following the confirmation that the infant has an adequate urinary stream

  E result in generally poor prognosis

(Answers overleaf)

11.1 **B D E**
An understanding of the anatomical and physiological
development of the kidney explains how young infants are more
vulnerable to fluid and electrolyte stress. The nephritogenic zone
of the outer cortex is active up to 36 weeks gestation, and the
newborn term infant has the definitive complement of
approximately 1 million nephrons in each kidney.
   Renal vascular resistance is high in the newborn and there is a
fourfold increase in fractional renal blood flow in the first year.
The GFR of the term infant is low compared to the adult, quoted
inulin clearance being 26–60 ml/min per 1.73 m^2 surface area.
Term infants are efficient at maintaining sodium balance on a
low intake but are susceptible to salt overload and
hypernatraemia. After water deprivation the newborn can
concentrate urine to 600–700 mmol/kg compared to the adult,
above 1200 mmol/kg.

11.2 **A C E**
Renal agenesis, renal dysplasia and infantile polycystic kidney
result in severe oligohydramnios and a characteristic pattern of
secondary features, including the Potter facies, redundant skin,
limb deformities and pulmonary hypoplasia. Approximately 40%
of infants with this syndrome complex are stillborn and the
remainder rarely survive beyound 2 days, death being due to
either respiratory or renal failure. A genetic basis has not been
fully defined but bilateral renal agenesis may represent severe
expression of a dominantly inherited gene which in milder
expression causes unilateral renal agenesis, and other renal tract
malformations. Parents and siblings should be screened by
ultrasound.

11.3 **A C**
In modern obstetric and paediatric practice, the majority of
cases are detected early. Bladder decompression procedures
have been developed for late fetal application, but these are
seldom justified as the majority of infants have a good outcome
if dealt with promptly after birth, and before the superimposition
of urinary infection and metabolic decompensation.
Confirmation of a good urinary stream should be a routine
component of assessing male infants. However, some infants
with severe obstruction have such fully developed detrusor
hypertrophy that they are able to produce an acceptable stream.

11.4 Urinary tract infection
   A has a prevalence of 2–3% in girls
   B requires renal tract imaging only after two or more infections have been confirmed
   C is associated with vesicoureteric reflux in more than 20% of children investigated
   D requires microbiological confirmation before selection of antibacterial therapy
   E is linked to constipation

11.5 Haematuria has a recognized association with
   A respiratory infection
   B hypercalciuria
   C haemolytic anaemia
   D pelviureteric junction obstruction
   E rifampicin treatment

11.6 Acute glomerulonephritis
   A is specifically related to prior group A β-haemolytic streptococcal infection
   B results in significant oliguria in the majority of cases
   C is a recognized cause of headache and convulsions
   D is an indication for long-term penicillin prophylaxis
   E results in hypocomplementaemia

11.7 Recognized features of Henoch Schönlein purpura include
   A a maculopapular skin rash over the buttocks
   B urticarial lesions
   C prolonged partial thromboplastin time
   D haematuria
   E generalized lymphadenopathy

(Answers overleaf)

11.4   **A C E**
Efforts to reduce the incidence and severity of renal scarring
need to be directed at prompt diagnosis and effective early
management of urinary tract infection in infants and young
children. Vesicoureteric reflux has been found in 35–40% of
children with urinary infection, and scarring arises in around a
third of those with reflux. Early antibacterial therapy can arrest
and prevent the development of scarring. This requires a low
threshold for considering urinary infection especially in infants
and young children with non-specific symptoms, adequate
sample collection, and immediate antibacterial treatment while
awaiting microbiological confirmation. In a recent retrospective
study, 50 of 52 children with bilateral scarring and reflux had
been ill-served by delays in diagnosis and treatment.
   A family history of vesicoureteric reflux, or fetal ultrasound
evidence of renal tract dilation, provide the opportunity for
evaluation and preventative measures before infection occurs.

11.5   **A B D**
Frank haematuria is relatively rare in childhood and red urine
may have an innocent explanation such as ingestion of some
confectinary dyes or drugs, notably rifampicin. Microscopic
haematuria has a broad range of aetiologies both within and
outside the renal tract. It is also easy for the urine to be
contaminated by blood from the external genital area or from
menses. Sensitive stick urinalysis may indicate transient
haematuria after vigorous excercise or during coincidental
febrile illness.

11.6   **C E**
Acute glomerulonephritis can also be a sequel to a range of viral
illnesses, e.g. varicella and mumps. It is also reported following
infection by group C strains of streptococcus.
   The majority of affected children have a mild illness
recognized because of smoky urine but without oliguria. Fluid
retention and hypertension in those children with oliguria can
result in an encephalopathic presentation.

11.7   **A B D**
Henoch Schönlein purpura refers to a pattern of self-limiting
vasculitis, most commonly encountered in childhood. The rash,
characteristically incorporating a haemorrhagic component, is
typically distributed over extensor surfaces. The urticarial
element may be generalized or localized producing, e.g. massive
oedema of scalp or scrotum. Nephritis is frequent and usually
insignificant. A small percentage, less than 5% and more
commonly older children, develop progressive
glomerulonephritis.

11.8 Nephrotic syndrome in childhood

- A is accepted as being the consequence of glomerular immune complex dispostion
- B is most frequent between ages 1 and 5 years
- C is a recognized cause of acute abdominal pain
- D requires prompt diuretic therapy during the phase of oedema formation
- E relapses in less than 10% of those who demonstrate a rapid complete response to corticosterod therapy at the primary episode

11.9 Recognized causes of acute renal failure in childhood include

- A verotoxin-producing *Escherichia coli* infection
- B insulin-dependent diabetes
- C remission induction therapy in acute leukaemia
- D neurogenic bladder
- E inappropriate antidiuretic hormone secretion

11.10 Undescended testes

- A are most frequent when cremasteric contraction is at its maximum between ages 2 and 8 years
- B are developmentally normal in the majority of cases operated on in early childhood
- C are palpable in the superficial inguinal pouch in approximately two-thirds of patients
- D are more susceptible to trauma
- E are more susceptible to torsion

(Answers overleaf)

11.8   **B C**
A wide range of immune function abnormalities have been
reported in minimal change nephrotic syndromes but none has
been generally accepted as causative. Whatever the
pathogenesis, there is growing evidence of disruption to the
glycosaminoglycans and associated negative charge sites within
the glomerular basement membrane.
The child with evolving oedema is potentially at risk from a
contracting intravascular volume. Injudicious use of diuretics can
aggravate circulatory collapse and secondary renal failure.
Approximately 75% of initially steroid-sensitive children will
relapse. The prognosis for such children is generally excellent
and it is worth remembering that the introduction of first
penicillin (1940s) and subsequently corticosteroids (1950s)
reduced the mortality rate from 40% to around 5%.

11.9   **A C D**
Urine output below 1 ml/kg/hour is insufficient to secrete solute
output and requires prompt investigation to establish whether
the cause is prerenal (circulatory insufficiency), renal or postrenal.
One of the commonest cause of renal failure in young children
is haemolytic uraemic syndrome linked to infections with certain
strains of *E. coli*.
Intensive tumour lysis strategies carry the risk of overloading
the kidneys with uric acid at a time when they are also subjected
to direct nephrotoxic effects. It is therefore essential to ensure a
high urine flow rate.
A neurogenic bladder is just one cause of obstructive uropathy
that needs to be excluded by clinical review and an early renal tract
ultrasound examination. Chronic renal failure has been reported
after 15–20 years diabetes duration in up to 40% of patients.
Fortunately, current patient cohorts appear to have a lower
prevalence. Acute renal failure is not a recognized complication of
diabetes and an alternative explanation must be sought.
Inappropriate ADH release complicates a range of disorders
from meningitis to bronchiolitis. It results in an expanded
extracellular volume with hyponatraemia; the urine is
inappropriately concentrated with an elevated sodium content.

11.10 **B C D**
An undescended testis is one that cannot be made to reach the
bottom of the scrotum. Approximately two-thirds are situated in the
superficial inguinal pouch and are therefore palpable in the groin. The
retractile testis can be manipulated to the bottom of the scrotum
despite starting as high as the superficial inguinal pouch. The
cremasteric muscle responsible for retractility is especially active
between ages 2 and 8 years, and hence the value of documenting
early infancy testicular descent in the parent-held record.
The majority of undescended testes start as being normal, and the
aim of early orchidopexy is to ensure intact spermatogenesis and to
prevent dysplasia. Undescended testes are at risk of trauma as they
lie adjacent to the pubic tubercle; they are less prone to torsion.

11.11 The following statements are true of inguinal hernias and hydroceles

A   over half of inguinal hernias detected at the newborn examination are self correcting and herniotomy should be delayed for 6 months

B   inguinal hernias are rarely irreducible in young infants

C   isolated scrotal hydroceles detected in the first 6 months of life should be treated conservatively

D   a spontaneously developing hydrocele in a schoolboy requires operative management

E   bilateral inguinal hernias in a girl may be associated with the 46 XY chromosome karyotype

11.12 Torsion of the testis

A   is less common than torsion of a testicular appendage

B   is caused by a torsion of the spermatic cord

C   is unlikely unless there was sudden onset of scrotal pain

D   may be adequately managed by non-operative untwisting of the gonad

E   is frequently associated with a bilateral anomaly of tunica vaginalis attachment to the cord

(Answers overleaf)

11.11 **C D E**

All inguinal hernias require surgical repair and the younger the child the more urgent the need. Irreducibility is a common complication in young infants and carries a high risk of testicular or bowel ischaemia.

Hydroceles which are present at or develop soon after birth may resolve spontaneously due to the normal obliteration of the processus vaginalis. In the older boy, testicular tumours may present as a hydrocele, hence the need for prompt exploration. The testicular feminization syndrome may manifest itself as bilateral inguinal hernias sometimes containing testes. Other than this presentation, it is unusual for this syndrome to present in childhood.

11.12 **A B E**

Torsion of a testicular appendage is the most common cause of acute scrotal pain (60%), followed by torsion of the testis, or to be more precise the spermatic cord (30%). The onset of scrotal pain may be gradual or intermittent and this can lead to delay in recognition.

Urgent scrotal exploration is mandatory whenever there is a risk of testicular torsion. The spermatic cord is untwisted and both testes are anchored to avoid later torsion.

12. Blood

12.1 Haemoglobin
- **A** at 40 weeks gestation is 70–75% HbF
- **B** at 40 weeks gestation is 20–25% HbA$_2$
- **C** after age 3 is over 98% HbA
- **D** after age 3 years is approximately 10% HbF
- **E** in β-thalassaemia minor contains elevated HbF and HbA$_2$

12.2 Iron-deficiency anaemia
- **A** may be prevented by the promotion of milk intake
- **B** contributes to more significant anaemia in infants who are breast rather than formula fed for the first 6 months
- **C** is associated with a higher incidence of early learning problems
- **D** is confirmed by demonstrating elevation of serum ferritin concentration
- **E** increases susceptibility to infection

12.3 Hereditary spherocytosis
- **A** is inherited as an autosomal dominant condition
- **B** may be confirmed by paper electrophoresis of whole blood
- **C** may cause severe jaundice in the newborn period
- **D** may be complicated by abrupt exacerbations of anaemia due to transient erythroid hypoplasia
- **E** is an indication for splenectomy in the first 3 years of life

12.4 Glucose-6-phosphate dehydrogenase deficiency
- **A** is inherited as a sex-linked condition
- **B** is not clinically manifest in girls
- **C** causes drug-induced haemolysis
- **D** is an indication for splenectomy
- **E** is more pronounced in mature red blood cells

(Answers overleaf)

12.1 **A C E**
After infancy normal haemoglobin consists of 98–99% HbA
($\alpha_2\beta_2$) with less than 2% HbF ($\alpha_2\gamma_2$) and less than 3% HbA2
($\alpha_2\delta_2$). At term HbF makes up 70–75% and it is largely replaced
by HbA by age 6 months. An appreciation of changing
haemoglobin is relevant to neonatal haemoglobinopathy
screening programmes as well as to the investigation of
anaemia, failure to thrive and pre-operative assessment of at-risk
racial groups.

12.2 **C E**
Dietary imbalance with delayed weaning and too great a
dependence on cow's milk is a common cause of iron
deficiency. Unfortified cow's milk contains little iron (0.5 mg/l)
and gastrointestinal sensitivity to cow's milk proteins may
provoke occult blood loss. Although breast milk contains little
more iron (1.5 mg/l), it is better absorbed and iron deficiency is
uncommon.
   Iron deficiency is more prevalent among inner city
populations and reflects poor nutritional understanding as much
as deprivation. Affected children are susceptible to a range of
adverse influences but recent carefully controlled studies
support the belief that iron deficiency depresses learning
function.

12.3 **A C D**
Although inherited as an autosomal dominant, parents may be
free of clinical features. Measurement of osmotic fragility will
confirm the diagnosis. Electrophoresis demonstrates normal
haemoglobin.
   Haemolytic and hypoplastic episodes both contribute to
anaemia. These crises are provoked by fever, and are manifest
by malaise, fever and abdominal pains.
   Splenectomy is the treatment of choice but is delayed until
the child is aged at least 4 years. Young splenectomized children
are vulnerable to septicaemia.

12.4 **A C E**
G6PD deficiency is transmitted as an incompletely dominant
sex-linked condition. Most males show complete expression but
females less so; among American blacks the prevalence in
males is 15% and in females is 2%.
   It is essential to inform affected persons of the drugs which
may provoke haemolysis. Haemolytic crises are self-limiting
because young red cells contain sufficient enzyme to avoid
damage. There is no place for splenectomy.

12.5   Sickle cell disease

    A is associated with increased polymerization of deoxygenated haemoglobin

    B is a recognized cause of prolonged neonatal jaundice

    C increases susceptibility to infection with encapsulated bacteria

    D is a cause of childhood stroke (cerebrovascular disease)

    E is conventionally managed by regular blood transfusions

12.6   β-thalassaemia major

    A is associated with a relative excess of β-globin molecules

    B results in a blood film exhibiting hypochromic, microcytic red cells

    C produces a generalized osteoporosis

    D is commonly associated with a reduced serum iron

    E results in delayed puberty

12.7   Haemophilia

    A does not cause a coagulation disturbance in the newborn infant

    B lacks a positive family history in one-third of affected boys

    C causes a prolonged bleeding time

    D causes a prolonged partial thromboplastin time (a test of the intrinsic coagulation pathway)

    E results from the synthesis of biologically inactive factor VIII (AHG)

(Answers overleaf)

12.5 **A C D**
Sickle cell disease is compatible with reasonable general health and growth, particularly if it is diagnosed in infancy so that appropriate precautions can be planned. Progressive splenic dysfunction makes affected children susceptible to overwhelming pneumococcal infection so that they should be given pneumococcal vaccine and prophylactic penicillin. There are several different types of potential crisis but the most threatening is cerebral infarction which occurs in approximately 8%. A stroke may complicate fever, dehydration or another crisis but it may also occur without obvious warning. There is a high risk of recurrence and this provides an accepted indication for a chronic transfusion programme to keep the sickle haemoglobin at less than 30%. Regular transfusions are not part of a conventional treatment plan for the majority of patients.

12.6 **B C E**
β-thalassaemia genes result in reduced synthesis of β-globin chains and therefore HbA_1. There is a compensatory increase in HbF and HbA_2. The result is ineffective erythropoiesis and chronic haemolysis. Thalassaemia is readily distinguished from iron deficiency by the finding of elevated serum iron. Iron therapy is contraindicated especially as the necessary transfusion programme creates iron overload and organ damage. The transfusion strategy is aimed at improving bone and general growth. Delayed puberty is a consistent feature, arising from chronic ill health, iron deposition in endocrine organs, and possibly as a side-effect of desferrioxamine leaching of zinc and other trace metals.

12.7 **B D E**
Factor VIII (AHG) does not cross the placenta and severe haemophilia may manifest itself in the neonatal period, especially if provoked by circumcision.
  Approximately one-third of haemophiliacs have no family history, either because it has arisen as a new mutation or because the mother is one of a long line of carriers without symptomatic male relatives.
  A history, such as bleeding for more than 24 hours after dental extraction, and a prolonged partial thromboplastin time suggest haemophilia. The next step is specific assay of factor VIII (AHG).
  Haemophilia results from the synthesis of a biologically inactive AHG. This abnormal peptide may be measured by immunoassay and provides a means of confirming carrier status.

12.8 Thrombocytopenia has a recognized association with
A   Henoch Schönlein purpura
B   septicaemia
C   rubella
D   Von Willebrand disease
E   portal hypertension

12.9 Recognized causes of rectal bleeding in infancy include
A   necrotizing enterocolitis
B   cow's milk protein intolerance
C   α1-antitrypsin deficiency
D   fissure-in-ano
E   giant haemangioma not involving the intestine

12.10 The following are valid associations in children with hypochromic anaemia
A   a normal serum ferritin and an elevated HbA_2 point to β-thalassaemia minor
B   a low ferritin and a normal HbA_2 exclude β-thalassaemia minor
C   a low ferritin points to iron deficiency
D   a raised ferritin and normal haemoglobin electrophoresis point to anaemia of a chronic inflammatory disorder
E   a dimorphic blood film is consistent with a recent blood transfusion

(Answers overleaf)

12.8   **B C E**
Thrombocytopenia may result from reduced platelet production caused by specific or generalized marrow failure, or from increased destruction. The commonest cause of the latter is a transient immune-mediated process. Viral infection may provoke either marrow failue or abnormally rapid destruction. Septicaemia is commonly complicated by disseminated intravascular coagulation and secondary thrombocytopenia. Hypersplenism is a further cause of thrombocytopenia and pancytopenia. It is important to differentiate abnormal bleeding or purpura due to other causes, e.g. faulty capillary endothelium as in Henoch Schönlein purpura, or defective platelet function as in Von Willebrand disease.

12.9   **A B C D E**
Minor degrees of rectal bleeding are common in healthy infants and can be explained by the swallowing of maternal blood from a cracked nipple or because of a fissure. Rectal bleeding and abdominal distension in a low birthweight infant raise the threat of evolving necrotizing enterocolitis. Ulcerative colitis provoked by cow's milk feeds is well described in infancy.

Early onset haemorrhagic disease of the newborn is closely linked to deficiency of vitamin K-induced coagulation factors (II, VII, IX and X). Late onset haemorrhagic disease, occuring in infants older than 2 weeks and in spite of routine vitamin K prophylaxis, suggests underlying liver disease such as that caused by α1-antitrypsin deficiency. Giant haemangiomas may consume platelets and cause a generalized bleeding disorder (Kasabach-Merritt syndrome).

12.10 **A C D E**
Ferritin measurement is a widely available parameter by which to assess tissue iron reserves. Relative iron deficiency is common in children and hence the wide limits of the normal range, 20–300 μg/l. Given the frequency of iron deficiency it is reasonable to assume that all children with an otherwise unexplained hypochromic anaemia will benefit from a course of oral iron. Haemoglobinopathies need to be considered in non-white children. β-thalassaemia minor is usually identified by electrophoresis showing increased HbA_2 (range 3.5–10%) and HbF (range 2–8%). However, affected children may also be iron deficient with a relatively depressed and hence normal HbA_2 (2–3.5%). If in doubt treat with iron for 3 months and repeat the electrophoresis so as to avoid inappropriate long-term iron therapy as well as to provide counselling.

13. Malignancy

13.1 Acute lymphatic leukaemia
A has a peak incidence between age 10 and 15 years
B may present without lymphoblasts being detected in peripheral blood
C has a better prognosis if the initial white blood cell count is less than $10 \times 10^9/l$
D is more frequent in children previously exposed to Epstein-Barr virus
E is consistent with a 5-year survival of greater than 60%

13.2 Acute lymphoblastic leukaemia is recognized as a cause of
A pleural effusion
B squint
C epistaxis
D diabetes insipidus
E polyarthritis

13.3 Nephroblastoma (Wilms tumour)
A frequently presents as an asymptomatic abdominal mass
B usually occurs in children aged under 5 years
C results in a mass which characteristically crosses the midline
D typically results in tumour-associated calcification visible on X-ray
E commonly presents with lung metastases

13.4 Neuroblastomas
A usually present as the result of increasing abdominal distension
B may present with limb pain
C produce hepatomegaly
D have a worse prognosis in children aged under 2 years
E metastasize to bone marrow

(Answers overleaf)

13.1   **B C E**
Acute lymphatic leukaemia (ALL) accounts for 85% of childhood
leukaemia and occurs throughout childhood with a peak around
5 years. The majority have conspicuous peripheral blood
lymphoblasts but in some children the lymphoblasts will only be
revealed by marrow examination. A low peripheral WBC is a
good prognostic factor; a count above 50 × 10^9/l, CSF
involvement, and a panel of cell markers are factors which
indicate a poorer prognosis and the need for intensified therapy.

13.2   **A B C D E**
Acute leukaemia is the great mimic of childhood practice.

13.3   **A B E**
The majority of nephroblastomas present in young children,
60% before age 3 and occasionally at birth. The abdominal
mass is often asymptomatic and may be discovered by accident
or on palpation during a routine health check. The mass is
usually unilateral, hard and has a smooth or gently lobulated
surface. They vary considerably in size; the largest may occupy
half the abdominal cavity but, unlike neuroblastomas, they tend
not to cross the midline. Tumour-associated calcification is a
feature of neuroblastomas. Metastases are common at
diagnosis, 40%, but if amenable to surgery or radiotherapy, they
do not deny the possibility of cure.

13.4   **B C E**
Neuroblastomas have a varied pattern of presentation reflecting
the range of abdominal and extra-abdominal primary sites,
compounded by almost inevitable metastases. The tumour load
and metastases results in malignant 'malaise', irritability, bone
pain, neurological signs, etc. The abdominal mass commonly
crosses the midline and may be difficult to distinguish from the
liver, which it may have invaded.
   The overall survival figures are still poor, but are better in
children aged under 2 years. Some primary tumours mature into
benign ganglioneuromas; and a subgroup of infants experience
spontaneous resolution in spite of initial spread to skin, liver and
bone marrow. Current research is attempting to exploit the
observation that this tumour clearance may have an immune
basis.

13.5 Retinoblastoma

A seldom has genetic implications
B may present as a 'white' reflex, the appearance of the pupil when illuminated
C is a cause of strabismus
D does not metastasize beyond the orbit
E tumours are radiosensitive

13.6 Hand–Schuller–Christian disease (Histiocytosis X)

A is frequently situated in the skull
B may present with a persistently discharging ear
C results in sclerotic lesions on skull X-ray
D may cause diabetes insipidus
E has a uniformly poor prognosis

13.7 The following are associated with an increased frequency of childhood malignancy

A trisomy 21
B corticosteroid therapy
C ataxia telangiectasia
D immune deficiency syndromes
E neurofibromatosis

13.8 Recognized complications of childhood cranial radiotherapy include

A learning problems
B growth hormone deficiency
C inappropriately early puberty
D second tumour induction
E deafness

(Answers overleaf)

13.5 **B C E**
Genetic counselling is essential: the risk to offspring of affected patients is 50% in the familial, bilateral type and 5–10% in the unilateral sporadic type.
Presenting features include a 'white' reflex, strabismus, glaucoma and proptosis.
The tumour spreads along the optic nerve and associated subarachnoid space, and may seed via the CSF. Distant extracranial metastases also occur, usually as a late event.

13.6 **A B D**
The classic triad comprises multiple rarefying lesions in membrane bones, exophthalmos and diabetes insipidus. Current usage associates it with the intermediate category of Histiocytosis X in which there is dissemination to both bone and soft tissue.
Prognosis is unpredictable; the outcome may be excellent especially if lesions are restricted to bone.

13.7 **A C D E**
Most human cancers aggregate in families and genetic susceptibility is especially relevant in the young. Recent advances in molecular genetics have established familial cancer phenotypes and opened up the possibility for screening techniques. An example of a cloned gene is p53 for the Li–Fraumeni syndrome, a dominantly inherited condition leading to early onset breast, adrenal and other tumours. Other examples are RBI for hereditary retinoblastoma, WT1 for some Wilms tumours, NF1 for neurofibromatosis type 1, and APC for familial adenomatous polyposis. Screening for genetic susceptibility to cancer will raise challenging social and ethical issues.

13.8 **A B C D**
Cranial radiotherapy is most frequently used as prophylaxis for acute lymphoblastic leukaemia (ALL), and as direct therapy in cranial tumours. The increasing survival of children with ALL has focused attention on the early and late side-effects of this treatment as these may detract from the quality of life. Neuropsychological sequelae are well recognized but have been difficult to define against a background of threatening disease and co-existent chemotherapy. Children aged under 2 years are especially vulnerable, and both radiation dose and fractionation can be modified to reduce damage.
Radiotherapy disrupts the neuronal integration responsible for the control of growth hormone secretion and the onset of puberty. The pubertal growth spurt may be depressed and limit final height. An early puberty can be an additional problem, especially in girls.
Radiation-induced second tumours are well documented. A survey of survivors of ALL has shown a 7-fold excess of all tumours and a 20-fold excess of CNS tumours; children under age 5 were especially liable to the latter.

14. Growth

14.1 **A 6-week-old boy has a head circumference of 41.5 cm (above the 98th centile). The following favour a conservative approach to management**
   A   father's head circumference is 59 cm (above the 98th centile)
   B   a palpable post-auricular fontanelle
   C   a lax anterior fontanelle
   D   a sun-setting eye sign
   E   an intracranial bruit

14.2 **Hydrocephalus is a recognized complication of**
   A   intraventricular haemorrhage
   B   Arnold-Chiari malformation
   C   benign intracranial hypertension
   D   achondroplasia
   E   megalocephaly

14.3 **Plagiocephaly**
   A   is a postural deformity
   B   is most noticeable in the early postnatal period
   C   is associated with unilateral shortening of the sternomastoid
   D   is associated with microcephaly
   E   is associated with ear malformation

(Answers overleaf)

14.1   **A C**

The majority of large heads are familial, and measurement of the parents' head circumference is important. Innocent large heads will follow a growth centile which is parallel to the normal. Increasing deviation is always a cause for concern.

The post-auricular fontanelle is not normally palpable. Suspect hydrocephalus if it accommodates a finger tip. Hydrocephalus should be diagnosed before secondary symptoms and signs such as sun-setting eyes arise.

A loud bruit suggests an intracranial arteriovenous malformation. Soft bruits are however common in normal infants.

14.2   **A B D**

Hydrocephalus refers to the abnormal accumulation of fluid within the ventricular system; the fluid is usually under increased pressure. Post-haemorrhagic hydrocephalus is relatively common in low birthweight infants. The Arnold–Chiari malformation is often associated with spina bifida, and refers to the downward displacement of the medulla oblongata and cerebellar tonsils through the foramen magnum. This displacement or adjacent adhesions block CSF flow.

Benign intracranial hypertension implies raised intracranial pressure due neither to inflammation nor a space-occupying lesion. The ventricles are usually normal or small on cranial CT examination. Bony deformities at the base of the skull in achondroplasia may result in hydrocephalus. Children affected by achondroplasia have relatively large skull vaults anyway and this additional problem may be overlooked.

Megalocephaly refers to brain growth at or above the upper limits of normal, and not to disturbed CSF flow.

14.3   **A C**

Plagiocephaly is a common early postural deformity in which one half of the skull is displaced forward compared to the other, producing a prominent brow on one side and flattened ipsilateral occiput. This has been descriptively termed the 'parallelogram' skull. Although it may be present at birth, it is often more conspicuous after the first month, reflecting the tendency for infants to prefer to rotate their heads to one side. There may be an underlying reason for restricted neck movement, e.g. a shortened sternomastoid. The more severe end of the plagiocephaly spectrum can cause family anxiety. Simple examination will readily distinguish this innocent condition from the rare premature fusion of a coronal suture.

14.4   The anterior fontanelle
  A   rarely closes before age 6 months in normal infants
  B   rarely closes after age 15 months in normal infants
  C   shows delayed closure in rickets
  D   is normally pulsatile
  E   shows delayed closure in cleidocranial dysostosis

14.5   The following are recognized indications for referring a short child for specialist assessment
  A   height consistently following the 2nd centile
  B   height in late childhood crossing the 9–25th centile channel to the 2–9th centile channel
  C   height velocity of a 3 year old below 5 cm per year
  D   height on the 5th centile compared to midparental height at 75th centile
  E   adolescent behaviour problems linked to short stature

14.6   Achondroplasia
  A   is inherited as an autosomal dominant condition
  B   occurring in the first child of normal parents indicates a 1:2 risk of a subsequently affected child
  C   causes disproportionate short stature
  D   primarily affects membranous bones
  E   may be complicated by spinal cord compression

14.7   Typical features of congenital growth hormone deficiency include
  A   reduced fetal growth
  B   susceptibility to hypoglycaemia
  C   diminished subcutaneous fat
  D   small genitalia
  E   delayed skeletal maturation

(Answers overleaf)

14.4 **C D E**
Anterior fontanelles in normal infants show considerable
variation in size, shape and time of closure. Closure may occur
between 4 and 26 months; 90% between 7 and 19 months.
Early or delayed closure is of little significance if head growth is
normal and it is an isolated finding. The normal fontanelle is
pulsatile, a useful sign when attempting to differentiate between
the innocent bulging fontanelle of a crying infant and the fixed
bulging due to elevated intracranial pressure.

14.5 **C D E**
The interpretation of a child's growth depends on accurate
measurement, adequate record keeping preferably on parent-
held health records, and correct use of appropriate national
growth standards. The key issues are whether the child has
growth failure rather than just short stature, and a stature
consistent with parental heights. The UK cross-sectional
standards have been updated in 1994 and incorporate guidance
on derivation of mid-parental centile and target centile range.
   It is relatively common for a prepubertal child's height to
cross downwards across one of the main centiles; this is
unlikely to be pathological unless there are other suspicious
features.
   Constitutional delay of growth and puberty is common
especially in boys, and its social and emotional implications may
warrant endocrine intervention to accelerate growth and sexual
maturation.

14.6 **A C E**
Achondroplasia is inherited as a highly penetrant autosomal
dominant condition but 80% arise as sporadic mutations, and
for these families the risk of recurrence is very low.
   Achondroplasia is the commonest cause of short limbed
dwarfism. Cartilaginous bones are involved, notably of the
limbs, face and base of the skull. Relative narrowing of the
foramen magnum may lead to spinal cord compression.

14.7 **B D E**
The majority of infants with congenital growth hormone
deficiency are of normal size at birth and appear to grow
normally during the first months of infancy. Tissue growth
factors other than pituitary growth hormone are more relevant
to growth in fetal and early postnatal growth. Reduced muscle
mass but increased skinfold thickness is typical. Growth
hormone has an additive effect with testosterone on penile
growth. Infant boys with micropenis and hypoglycaemia should
be investigated for congenital hypopituitarism.

14.8 The following are recognized features of Turner syndrome

A otitis media with effusion
B accelerated skeletal maturation
C coarctation of the aorta
D pulmonary stenosis
E low hair line

14.9 Growth hormone (GH)

A controls height velocity as the result of alterations in the frequency of pulsatile secretion
B is present in plasma in a complex mixture of molecular variants
C acts on hepatocytes to promote the release of insulin-like growth factor
D deficiency is most commonly due to a fault in the growth hormone gene cluster
E underproduction is the basis of small stature in African pygmies

(Answers overleaf)

14.8 **A C E**
Turner syndrome needs to be considered in any girl who is
inappropriately short for her parental height. All too often the
diagnosis is not considered or is dismissed because the girl
does not show the more conspicuous features highlighted by
standard textbooks. Girls may attend ENT, eye, cardiac or even
paediatric clinics without the diagnosis being made. The
syndromatic features may be subtle and there has to be a low
threshold for performing a karyotype.

A high arched palate is linked with eustachian dysfunction and
impaired middle ear ventilation so that conductive deafness is
common, adding to other learning difficulties. Delayed skeletal
maturation is common and is accentuated by the lack of a
spontaneous pubertal growth spurt.

14.9 **B C**
Chromosome 17 contains the GH gene cluster made up of two
GH genes and three placental lactogens. The principle GH is a
191 amino acid, 22 000 dalton product (22K), but this represents
only about half of the circulating GH forms found shortly after a
secretory burst. This biological complexity is further influenced
by GH binding proteins and the whole cocktail explains some of
the problems of plasma GH assays. GH secretion is an example
of a biological control system controlled by pulse amplitude.
The pulse periodicity is highly conserved.

The growth promoting effects of GH are largely dependent on
liver and other peripheral tissue derived insulin-like growth
factor-1 (IGF-1). African pygmies are not GH deficient but they
do have reduced GH-receptor activity.

The majority of GH deficiency is due to disordered pulsatile
secretion due to faults in the hypothalamo-pituitary axis.

15. Endocrine

15.1 The following findings are recognized as being within the spectrum of normal female development

   A fluctuating symmetrical breast development in the first 18 months of life
   B pubic hair growth from age 7 years
   C intermittent vaginal bleeding before breast development
   D height acceleration in parallel with breast bud formation
   E ultrasound appearance of multicystic ovaries

15.2 The following findings are recognized within the spectrum of normal male sexual development

   A advanced penile growth with testicular volumes of less than 4 ml
   B onset of puberty delayed beyond age 15 years
   C asymmetrical breast development in mid puberty
   D scanty pubic hair growth from age 6 years
   E bone age delay of 1.5 years at age 14 years

15.3 Recognized causes of delayed puberty include

   A anorexia nervosa
   B gluten enteropathy
   C ovarian dysgenesis
   D cranial radiotherapy
   E sodium valproate therapy

(Answers overleaf)

15.1 **A B D E**
Infants may have transient breast development in the neonatal period. It is also relatively common for there to be a self-limiting phase of symmetrical or asymmetrical breast growth between 6 months and 2 years. This isolated thelarche is not accompanied by pubic hair growth or by height acceleration, and appears to be associated with increased FSH but not LH secretion.

Isolated pubic hair growth, accompanied by modest growth acceleration, reflects the maturation of adrenal cortical androgen production.

Isolated menarche has been described but it is rare and a girl presenting with isolated vaginal bleeds requires careful assessment to exclude foreign body insertion, trauma including sexual abuse, or a local bleeding lesion, e.g. a tumour.

Height acceleration is an early component of the female puberty, increasing feet size is often remarked on.

Pelvic ultrasound has become a useful tool for evaluating female sexual maturation. Ovarian growth and follicle formation may be evident from age 6 years. A multicystic appearance is normal before the maturation of dominant follicles.

15.2 **C D E**
The accessibility of the testes for measurement, preferably with an orchidometer, allows for relatively easy clinical evaluation of male sexual maturation. The normal progression is for testicular enlargement beyond 4 ml to precede penile growth, and for testes to have reached 8–10 ml before height acceleration. Advancing sexual maturation which is discordant from testicular enlargement points to an alternative source of androgens, most probably from the adrenal cortex.

As a rule girls should have entered puberty by age 14 years, and boys by age 15 years, but interpretation of delay should take account of the whole tempo of childhood growth. It may be justified to investigate a younger boy if either anxiety or clinical features cause concern. Constitutional delay of growth and puberty is, however, common in boys, and it may be sufficient to base the diagnosis on a positive family history and appropriate bone age delay.

15.3 **A B C D**
Early onset anorexia nervosa is a well recognized cause of delayed puberty; it appears that at least some of the affected girls adopt self-starvation so as to delay the imposition of a mature sexual role. Children of both sexes with less florid nutritional problems may still suffer adolescent growth failure and delayed puberty.

Cranial irradiation for tumours or as prophylaxis in the management of acute lymphoblastic leukaemia may disturb neuroendocrine control, particularly of growth hormone and gonadotrophin secretion. The ultimate effect on the timing of puberty is unpredictable; it may be delayed or inappropriately early as judged against the rest of the child's growth.

15.4 The onset of sexual maturation
A   is dependent on activation of gonadotrophin releasing
    hormone (GnRH) secretion
B   is independent of nutritional status
C   is genetically determined
D   may be prematurely activated following cranial irradiation
E   is more susceptible to premature activation in boys
    compared to girls

15.5 In normal sexual differentiation
A   the Müllerian duct system is suppressed by a product of the
    testis
B   fallopian duct and uterine development is dependent on
    functioning ovaries
C   the persistence of the mesonephritic or Wolffian duct system
    is dependent on Leydig cell activity
D   the fetal pituitary gland is the dominant source of
    gonadotrophin
E   males have a postnatal surge of gonadotrophin and
    testosterone

15.6 Congenital adrenal hyperplasia presents with
A   hypospadias and impalpable gonads
B   hypokalaemia
C   precocious puberty in boys
D   palpable loin masses
E   vomiting in the second week of life

15.7 Congenital hypothyroidism
A   is usually the result of autosomal recessive inheritance
B   is amenable to detection by a specific and sensitive neonatal
    screening test
C   is usually associated with a goitre
D   is caused by maternal iodine deficiency
E   is associated with prolonged gestation

(Answers overleaf)

15.4   **A C D**
Puberty is the end result of sexual differentiation and maturation, the two phases being separated by the quiescent period of childhood. It is likely that the trigger to maturation is the end-result of both internal and external influences. As yet ill-defined maturational events in the brain remove inhibition from the GnRH pulse generator which in turn stimulates increased amplitude of LH and FSH secretion. Genetic influence is evident from the correlation of age of menarche within families. On average identical twins reach menarche within 2 months of one another compared to 8 months in non-identical twins. The integrity of neuronal mechanisms responsible for pubertal restraint may be disturbed by hypothalamic tumours, hydrocephalus, trauma and cranial irradiation. Early puberty is at least 5 times more common in girls than boys, and is far more likely to be innocent. Detailed cranial imaging is not justified in girls unless puberty is abnormal in its progression or is accompanied by suspicious features, e.g. the onset of headaches or a cranial nerve palsy.

15.5   **A C E**
In male fetuses the Müllerian duct system degenerates and vanishes between 9 and 11 weeks. This is the result of local diffusion of Müllerian inhibitory factor (MIF) from the testicular Sertoli cells. Persistence of the Mullerian system and its differentiation into fallopian ducts, uterus and upper vagina is dictated by the absence of testes, not by the presence of ovaries. On this basis girls with Turner syndrome have differentiated internal genitalia.
  Testosterone is essential for the conversion of the Wolffian ducts into male internal genitalia. Placental secretion of human chorionic gonadotrophin (HCG) is the dominant stimulus to Leydig cell production of testosterone during organogenesis.

15.6   **A C E**
The commonest variety, 21-hydroxylase deficiency, causes virilization of the female fetus so that the newborn may be confused with a cryptorchid boy. Hyponatraemia and hyperkalaemia are the hallmarks of a salt-losing crisis.
  The adrenal origin of precocious 'pseudo puberty' can be clinically suspected because the testes remain small.

15.7   **B D E**
Congenital hypothyroidism in areas where iodine deficiency is not endemic arises as a sporadic disorder of thyroid differentiation. The introduction of TSH measurement in neonatal screening programmes has been one of the success stories of preventative medicine. Despite minimal transplacental thyroxine transfer, the fetal brain is relatively protected until delivery but it is essential to introduce thyroxine replacement promptly after birth. It also has to be appreciated that infants have a high thyroxine requirement. Prolonged gestation is common in congenital hypothyroidism.

15.8   Juvenile or acquired hypothyroidism
   A   is most commonly due to autoimmune thyroiditis
   B   is an important cause of mental handicap
   C   causes severe delay of skeletal maturation
   D   is more prevalent in children with Down syndrome
   E   is linked to familial thyroglobulin deficiency

15.9   Maternal thyrotoxicosis
   A   may result in fetal tachycardia
   B   places the fetus at risk as the result of excessive placental
       transfer of free thyroxine
   C   is a contraindication to the use of thiouracil drugs, e.g.
       carbimazole
   D   may result in neonatal thyrotoxicosis lasting 2–3 months
   E   is an absolute contraindication to breastfeeding

15.10 Insulin-dependent diabetes mellitus (IDDM)
   A   is more likely to be associated with a positive family history
       than non-insulin-dependent diabetes
   B   shows concordance in less than 50% of identical twins
   C   can be reliably screened for using HLA antigen analysis
   D   can be reliably screened for using islet-cell antibody
       measurement
   E   occurs in 2–5% of the offspring of an affected parent

(Answers overleaf)

15.8   **A C D**
Traditionally this terminology has been reserved for children
presenting after age 2 years and without features of missed
congenital hypothyroidism. Autoimmune thyroiditis is the most
common cause; there may be a positive family history or the
child may have other autoimmune disturbance, e.g. diabetes.
Acquired hypothyroidism may impair school performance but
does not produce permanent intellectual damage. It is an
important diagnosis to consider in children presenting with short
stature or subnormal height velocity.
  Several studies have demonstrated an increased prevalence
of hypothyroidism in children and adults with Down syndrome.
Clinical recognition is a problem and there is a case for regular
biochemical screening of this 'at risk' population.

15.9   **A D**
Maternal thyrotoxicosis is relatively common and it places the
fetus at risk from stillbirth, premature labour and symptomatic
thyrotoxicosis either before or after delivery. Even mothers with
quiescent disease may produce combinations of stimulating and
blocking antibodies that interact with the fetal thyroid to produce
variable patterns of hypo- and/or hyperthyroidism. The task of
the obstetrician is to keep both mother and fetus euthyroid.
Approximately 1 in 80 of affected pregnancies results in fetal or
neonatal thyrotoxicosis. Carbimazole therapy directed at the
maternal thyroid must be of modest dosage in order to avoid
fetal goitre formation and hypothyroidism. Fetal tachycardia,
indicating thyrotoxicosis, is an indication for prescribing high
dosage carbimazole to mother but with thyroxine so that she is
not rendered hypothyroid.

15.10 **B E**
Genetic factors, in part linked to HLA-DR 3 and 4, determine
susceptibility to IDDM but there is a large environmental
component accounting for at least 80% of an individual's risk
status. The environmental contribution is emphasized by the
relatively low concordance in identical twins. The nature of
these external influences remains a mystery but there are clues
from the increased prevalence in Northern Europe, the secular
trend towards a higher incidence, and a positive correlation with
socio-economic status.
  Neither HLA typing nor islet-cell antibodies alone can reliably
identify at-risk individuals. We still need to identify additional
susceptibility areas in the genome and studies of multiplex
families are likely to throw light on this. Current research studies
of pre-diabetes rely on a combination of HLA typing,
measurement of both islet-cell antibodies and activated T-cells,
as well as determination of insulin secretory reserve.

15.11 The following are accepted components of modern diabetes management

A   restricting carbohydrates to less than 40% of dietary energy
B   child or parent responsibility for insulin dose adjustment
C   daily measurement of glycosuria
D   promoting a target glycosylated haemoglobin (HbA1$_c$) in the low normal range
E   annual retinal examination

15.12 Hypoglycaemia is a recognized complication of

A   Reye syndrome
B   prolonged febrile convulsions
C   congenital adrenal hyperplasia
D   phenylketonuria
E   inherited defects of fatty acid oxidation

15.13 Hyponatraemia and hyperkalaemia are recognized findings in

A   anterior pituitary failure
B   congenital adrenal hyperplasia
C   adrenal cortical failure
D   obstructive uropathy
E   inappropriate antidiuretic hormone secretion

(Answers overleaf)

15.11 **B E**

Attitudes to nutrition in diabetes have been revised as we have
recognized the potential hazards of carbohydrate restriction with
a resulting excessive reliance on fat. The broad principles are to
promote a healthy balanced diet in which carbohydrate should
make up 50–55% of the dietary energy with the majority of this
coming from complex sources.

Education and motivation are essential to a successful and
independent diabetic life. Families need to take control based on
adequate blood sugar profiles performed for their own decision
making rather than to placate doctors.

There is now compelling evidence that improved diabetic
control reduces late complications but there are also real
hazards due to hypoglycaemia, especially in the young. An
individual's target metabolic control needs to take account of
how readily good control can be achieved; this will be
influenced by residual endogenous insulin production, age,
duration of diabetes, social factors, etc. It might be realistic to
aim for a $HbA1_c$ within the normal mean plus 2–3 SD.

15.12 **A C E**

Prompt blood glucose determination is mandatory in any child
with unexplained impairment of consciousness or seizures.
Hypoglycaemia together with evidence of disturbed liver
function (elevated plasma ammonia, raised transaminases,
prolonged prothrombin time) suggests Reye syndrome, a
metabolic error or the effect of a liver toxin.

Adrenal and pituitary insufficiency, or insulin excess, are well
recognized causes of hypoglycaemia. The stress associated with
febrile convulsions usually results in temporary, modest
hyperglycaemia.

15.13 **B C D**

The combination of hyponatraemia and hyperkalaemia is one of
the 'red flag' warning signals of medicine, and points to either
disordered aldosterone synthesis or action, or to renal tubule
pathology. In an infant or child without features of renal disease
(urine microscopy and culture normal, normal renal tract
ultrasound) the focus must be on evaluating adrenal cortical
function with measurement of plasma cortisol, ACTH and
adrenal androgens (17OH-progesterone, androstenedione).

Anterior pituitary failure may lead to ACTH and cortisol
deficiency with the potential for hyponatraemia but not for
hyperkalaemia. The commonest cause of hyponatraemia in
hospitalized patients is inappropriate ADH secretion causing
expansion of the extracellular volume and secondary natriuresis.

16. Skin

16.1 In the newborn the following cutaneous conditions are innocent and self-limiting
A milia
B erythema toxicum
C scalded skin syndrome
D harlequin colour change
E subcutaneous fat necrosis

16.2 The following are recognized causes of napkin rash
A seborrhoeic dermatitis
B Tinea corporis
C candidiasis
D atopic dermatitis
E intertrigo

16.3 Atopic eczema
A usually arises within the first month of life
B resolves by 2 years of age in at least 50% of children
C is an indication for a cow's milk free diet
D contraindicates triple immunization
E contraindicates BCG vaccination

16.4 Skin testing in allergic disorders
A is based on the detection of mast cell-fixed IgE antibodies
B has high specificity for patients with clinical evidence of allergy
C has high sensitivity for patients with clinical evidence of allergy
D has good correlation with double-blind food provocation challenges
E give false-negative results after therapy with H_1-receptor antagonists

(Answers overleaf)

16.1   **A   B   D   E**
Milia are minute sebaceous retention cysts and appear as
yellow-white specks over the nose and face.
   Erythema toxicum is a benign rash but the sometimes
widespread macules, papules and pustules may cause alarm. It
usually occurs within the first 48 hours of life and may last from
hours to a few days. The infant remains well, and a Gram stain
of the pustular fluid reveals eosinophils and no bacteria.
   The scalded skin syndrome is caused by virulent
staphylococcal infection.
   The harlequin colour change is more common in low
birthweight infants and occurs while they are lying on their
sides. The dependent half becomes red and the superior half
pale, probably reflecting immaturity of the autonomic nervous
system.
   Fat necrosis is usually limited to small areas adjacent to bone
surfaces and may follow birth injury. It seldom causes cosmetic
problems.

16.2   **A   C   D   E**
The main causes of napkin area dermatitis are friction, low-
grade infection and ammonia exposure. The traumatized skin is
then vulnerable to a range of other disorders including
candidiasis, seborrhoeic dermatitis, atopic eczema and
psoriaform lesions.

16.3   **B   E**
Although atopic eczema is common after the second month of
life, it is very uncommon in the first month.
   Specific allergens can only rarely be incriminated in atopic
eczema and there is no place for the widespread introduction of
cow's milk free diets.
   BCG vaccination is potentially hazardous for these children but
there is no contraindication to triple immunization.

16.4   **A   E**
A weal and flare response to the introduction of an allergen into
the skin is based on the presence of mast cell-fixed antibodies,
predominantly IgE. Most authorities believe that skin tests have
a role in research but have limited application to clinical
practice. Positive skin tests occur in patients with no clinical
evidence of allergy and may persist after problems have
resolved. Over 15% of allergic subjects have negative skin tests.
Skin tests are a poor guide to modifying the diet or environment
of most allergic patients, and their limited value may be
modified by long duration anti-histamine agents.

16.5 Impetigo

    A is highly contagious
    B is usually secondary to a streptococcal sore throat
    C in an infant may be complicated by generalized exfoliation
    D usually commences on the scalp
    E is an indication for oral chlortetracycline therapy

16.6 Vascular malformations. The following statements are correct

    A strawberry naevi usually disappear spontaneously by the age of 5 years
    B a facial port-wine lesion has a recognized association with focal motor seizures
    C cystic hygromas seldom increase in size after birth
    D congenital pedal lymphoedema is a feature of Turner syndrome
    E extensive limb haemangiomas usually impair growth of underlying bone

16.7 The following are recognized associations

    A warts and papilloma virus
    B Molluscum contagiosum and Pityrosporum yeast
    C severe erosive stomatitis and Herpes simplex
    D Erythema infectiosum and human parvovirus B19
    E hand, foot and mouth vesicles and Coxsachie virus

16.8 The following skin-related disorders are inherited as autosomal dominant conditions

    A cavernous haemangioma
    B neurofibromatosis
    C ichthyosis vulgaris
    D tuberous sclerosis
    E congenital pedal lymphoedema

(Answers overleaf)

16.5 **A C**
School outbreaks have been traced to staphyloccal (phage type
71) contamination of communal football kits. The recommended
'cool' wash is insufficient to kill the organism. The nostrils and
perioral areas are the most frequent sites. Scalp involvement
suggests head lice infestation. Chlortetracycline may be used
topically: systemic use is contraindicated in the growing child as
it damages the developing dentition.

16.6 **A B D**
The Sturge–Weber syndrome comprises a facial port-wine
naevus, with angiomatous involvement of ipsilateral meninges.
The underlying cerebral cortex is either atrophic or scarred
because of calcification in the abnormal meningeal vessels.
Focal motor seizures and a contralateral hemiparesis are
frequent manifestations.
    Cystic hygromas are benign and multiloculated tumours of
lymphatic origin. They are most commonly situated in the neck
and they tend to increase in size, sometimes rapidly. Surgical
excision is usually necessary.
    Vascular naevi of a limb are more likely to cause overgrowth of
bone and soft tissues, the Klippel–Trenauney–Weber syndrome.

16.7 **A C D E**
There are at least 40 strains of human papilloma virus. Warts, which
are unusual before age 3 years, usually have a self-limiting course
with resolution paralleled by the emergence of cellular immunity.
    Molluscum contagiosum is due to a pox virus, and may
manifest as a single umbilicated pearly papule or in crops. They
resolve within a year.
    Erythema infectiosum produces a confluent erythematous
rash over the cheeks, hence 'slapped face disease', as well as
over the trunk.

16.8 **B C D**
Cavernous haemangiomas are sporadic localized growth disorders
of subcutaneous tissue, dermis and vascular components.
    Neurofibromatosis type 1 is an important dominant disorder
although around half of cases present as new mutations.
    Ichthyosis vulgaris is a common condition, 1 in 1000, causing
hyperkeratosis and scaling.
    Tuberous sclerosis is an autosomal dominant disease with a
high new mutation rate. It enters the differential diagnosis of
early onset epilepsy, especially infantile spasms and
developmental delay. In early life the skin signs are subtle areas
of hypopigmentation which may be revealed by examination
under a Wood's lamp. Other skin features emerge with age;
periungual fibromas, facial angiofibromas and a shagreen patch
of thickened soft skin over the lumbar area.
    Pedal lymphoedema in a female infant is suggestive of Turner
syndrome.

17. Bone and joint

17.1 **Pyogenic arthritis**
   A is usually secondary to spread of infection across the epiphyseal growth plate
   B is most commonly caused by *Staphylococcus pyogenes*
   C causes rapid destruction of articular cartilage
   D rarely involves the hip joint
   E must be confirmed by joint aspiration

17.2 **Polyarthritis is a recognized complication of infection by**
   A rubella
   B parvovirus
   C varicella
   D campylobacter
   E mumps

17.3 **Recognized cause of non-infectious arthritis in childhood include**
   A diabetes mellitus
   B penicillin sensitivity
   C leukaemia
   D hypermobility syndrome
   E haemoglobin SS

17.4 **Recognized features of Henoch Schönlein purpura include**
   A a self-limiting thrombocytopenia
   B symmetrical arthritis
   C localized oedema
   D the risk of intussusception
   E prominent lymphadenopathy

17.5 **Characteristic presenting features of juvenile chronic polyarthritis include**
   A a persistent fever
   B a macular rash
   C generalized lymphadenopathy
   D erythema marginatum
   E iridocyclitis

(Answers overleaf)

17.1 **B C E**
The growth plate is an effective barrier against infection, and it is only in joints such as the hip that the metaphysis, by lying within the capsule, can provide the primary septic focus.
Pus destroys articular cartilage. The latter has little capacity to regenerare and the joint may be permanently damaged.
The hip is at risk especially in infancy. Being a deep joint the signs are often overlooked.

17.2 **A B C D E**
Rubella arthritis is seen predominantly in adolescent and adult females. Parvovirus is increasingly recognized as a cause of transient arthritis in the older age group. Transient arthritis as a manifestation of immune-complex disturbance is a feature of several systemic viral infections, and it is important to consider this aetiology when investigating polyarthritis and suspected juvenile chronic arthritis.
Campylobacter and other bacterial gut infection may be associated with a number of extra-intestinal infections including arthritis, erythema nodosum and Guillain-Barré syndrome. Enteric associated arthritis are linked to a higher prevalence of the haplotype HLA-B27.

17.3 **B C D E**
The many causes of polyarthritis always provide a good test of an organized approach to differential diagnosis. Drug sensitivity is a common cause of arthralgia and arthritis. Arthritis-like symptoms may precede the recognition of leukaemia or neuroblastoma by months. Children with lax or hypermobile joints are prone to joint injury as well as delayed walking. Small joint pain related to microinfarcts is a common manifestation of sickle cell disease in young children.

17.4 **B C D**
Henoch Schönlein purpura is an acute immune-mediated vasculitis. The provoking factor is seldom defined. The characteristic rash is the usual clue to explain the accompanying arthritis, abdominal pain and nephritis. Massive local oedema may produce striking but transient distortion of scalp or scrotum.

17.5 **B C E**
The diagnosis of juvenile chronic polyarthritis (JCA) is based on clinical and not laboratory findings. While it is important to know the cardinal features, you must also appreciate that the systemic onset variety of JCA may have varied and misleading presentations, e.g. with abdominal pain or with fever and neck stiffness.

17.6 Osteomyelitis

  A presents most commonly in the epiphyseal plate of the lower femur or upper tibia
  B is consistent with extensive bone destruction in an afebrile neonate
  C requires confirmation by aspiration of the periosteum
  D is most commonly due to Group A streptococcal infection
  E is more common in children with sickle cell disease

17.7 Structural scoliosis

  A is normally apparent by age 5 years
  B is accompanied by vertebral rotation
  C is a frequent complication of muscular dystrophy
  D has a recognized association with congenital dislocation of the hip
  E is amenable to prevention by established screening programmes

17.8 Congenital dislocation of the hip

  A has an incidence of between 1 and 1.5 per 1000 live births in NW Europe
  B affects both sexes equally
  C is the probable outcome in the majority of hips in which a click is detected in the newborn period
  D may be confirmed at 1 month of age by an X-ray examination of the hip
  E persisting at the time of walking results in a gait in which the opposite knee is kept flexed

17.9 Perthes disease

  A is mainly a disorder of adolescent boys
  B results from avascular necrosis of the femoral head
  C typically results in greater discomfort than transient synovitis of the hip
  D causes a limitation of hip abduction in flexion
  E necessitates prolonged bedrest

17.10 Talipes equinovarus

  A indicates inward rotation of the heel
  B has an incidence of about 1 per 1000 live births
  C has a risk of recurrence in the same family of greater than 1 in 10
  D responds to manipulative therapy in approximately 60% of infants
  E is associated with myelomeningocele

(Answers overleaf)

17.6 **B E**
Osteomyelitis originates in bone adjacent to venous sinusoids of the metaphysis (not the epiphysis), and the lower femur and upper tibia are most at risk.

Osteomyelitis in the neonate may be a component of a severe septicaemic illness, but a more common presentation is in an afebrile infant who presents because of crying with movement, e.g. napkin changing. X-rays at presentation can show extensive bone destruction. In older children, X-rays are seldom diagnostic in the first 7–10 days and radioisotope bone scans play an important part in diagnosis. In suspected osteomyelitis blood cultures usually reveal the bacterial pathogen and there is seldom justification to drain the periosteum for diagnostic purposes. *Staphylococcus aureus* is the most frequent pathogen.

17.7 **B C**
The majority of structural scoliosis is idiopathic and becomes apparent in girls between ages 10 and 14 years. The curve is fixed and is accompanied by vertebral rotation and rib prominence. Screening methods aimed at assessing spinal curves and rib humps in forward bending positions are under scrutiny, but they have not yet been recognized as reliable, cost-effective procedures.

17.8 **A E**
Girls are affected more than boys, 6:1.

Careful screening of all newborn infants detects instability in between 1:80 and 1:120. All of these need to be reviewed by an experienced person but less than 10% are likely to have a true dislocation.

Hip X-rays are unhelpful before 4 months of age.

Hip instability and leg shortening in young children causes them to keep the foot of the affected leg flat on the ground so that the opposite knee has to be flexed.

17.9 **B D**
Perthes disease is most common between 4 and 10 years of age.

The clinical onset is often indistinguishable from transient synovitis. The limp is more notable that the discomfort.

This variable condition requires individual assessment and management. Those hips judged not to be at risk from deformity do not benefit from bedrest, calipers or surgery.

17.10 **A B D E**
The foot is inverted and supinated, and the forefoot adducted. The normal space between the medial malleolus and the navicular tubercle is diminished. The inheritance pattern is multifactorial with mixed genetic and environmental influences. The overall incidence is about 1 per 1000 live births but the incidence in first-degree relatives is 20-fold increased, amounting to a recurrence rate of 1 in 35.

18. Brain, cord, nerve and muscle

18.1 The following features are consistent with meningitis in young children

- A febrile convulsions
- B normal body temperature
- C cranial nerve palsy
- D mucopurulent nasal discharge
- E diarrhoea

18.2 The following CSF findings are consistent with bacterial meningitis

- A a clear appearance
- B more than 50 red blood cells per mm^3
- C glucose of 2.9 mmol/l compared with blood glucose 5.2 mmol/l
- D no detectable organisms on Gram stain
- E polymorphs 50 per mm^3

18.3 Aseptic meningitis may be caused by

- A adenovirus
- B listeria
- C Reye syndrome
- D candida
- E leukaemia

18.4 Herpes simplex encephalitis

- A rarely occurs in the absence of skin vesicles
- B typically results in an excess of CSF lymphocytes
- C requires brain biopsy before starting acyclovir therapy
- D may be reliably excluded by cranial CT scan appearance
- E is caused by primary infection with Herpes simplex type 2

(Answers overleaf)

18.1   **A B C D E**
The non-specific nature of meningitis-related signs and symptoms keeps all of us on our toes! Surveys suggest that between a quarter and a third of young children with meningitis present with a picture compatible with a simple febrile convulsion. However, the yield of bacterial meningitis from routine examination of CSF in children presenting with their first febrile convulsion is very low, only 1 in 300 in a Nottingham study.

18.2   **A B C D E**
Typically, bacterial meningitis produces clear-cut evidence on CSF examination but there are potential problems if, for example, the child has already received antibiotics, the lumbar puncture was traumatic or the CSF sample has been mishandled. In situations where the clinical picture is suggestive of a viral infection and aseptic meningitis, but where the CSF findings are equivocal, it may be justified to repeat the lumbar puncture after 12 hours. This serial observaton may confirm a shift from polymorphs to lymphocytes in the CSF, thus confirming viral meningitis. It is obviously wise to ensure that bacterial culture of the CSF samples is organized.

18.3   **A D E**
Aseptic meningitis is defined as the presence of meningeal signs, CSF pleocytosis and negative routine bacterial cultures. Routine cultures in the neonatal period must include prolonged culture for the slow-growing Listeria. The vast majority of cases are due to viral infection but there is an extensive list of possible aetiologies, including fungi, protozoa, chlamydia, rickettsia, chemical irritation, and malignancy.

18.4   **B E**
Herpes simplex type 1 is the commonest cause of sporadic encephalitis, but type 2 infection acquired in the neonatal period, and often by direct transmission from the maternal genital tract, may produce encephalitis as part of a disseminated infection. At least 70% of cases do not have skin lesions, and therefore there must be a low threshold for considering this diagnosis when a child presents with fever, fits, behavioural change and no other satisfactory explanation. EEG and CT scan may be consistent with Herpes encephalitis but their main role is in excluding other disorders, e.g. brain abscess or tumour. The CSF examination may be suggestive of viral infection but can contain increased polymorphs, red blood cells and have a decreased glucose. Brain biopsy is redundant and acyclovir treatment is justified whenever Herpes infection cannot be excluded. Polymerase chain reaction (PCR) testing for Herpes simplex is now an accessible tool in routine clinical practice.

18.5   The diagnosis of epilepsy

    A should not be based on the occurrence of a single brief generalized seizure

    B can be excluded by a normal EEG

    C can be based solely on an EEG showing localized abnormality

    D may be based on parents' history alone

    E justifies the child's exclusion from school swimming lessons

18.6   Complex partial (temporal lobe) seizures

    A always result in alteration of consciousness

    B are always linked to generalized tonic-clonic movements

    C are usually preceded by an aura

    D are rare in the first decade of life

    E are an indication for treatment with carbamazepine

(Answers overleaf)

18.5   **A   D**
Most authorities would avoid labelling a child as having epilepsy
after a single seizure following which there is full recovery.
Investigation and treatment are usually reserved for patients
who have a prolonged episode, an attack from which there is
incomplete recovery, or who have had two or more seizures
within a year.

About 15% of people with epilepsy never have EEGs showing
specific epileptiform discharges, and the description of an eye-
witness may be sufficient to make the diagnosis. Diagnosis
should not be based solely on EEG as between 10 and 15% of
the population have an 'abnormal' EEG.

A careful history is the key to correct diagnosis but it is not
infallable, either because non-epileptic seizures may resemble
epilepsy or because a parent chooses to fabricate evidence.
Always be prepared to reconsider the diagnosis, especially if
anticonvulsant treatment appears to be ineffective.

Epileptic children have to be protected from inappropriate
restriction and prejudice.

18.6   **A   C   E**
Partial seizures of complex symptomatology have by definition
an impairment or alteration of consciousness. Abnormal
discharges in the temporal lobe produce abnormal
manifestations of the lobe's normal function, which is to
integrate sensations. Auras may mimic the special senses or
involve somatic or visceral awareness. The complexity of the
aura may defy the ability of young children to describe them,
and hence under-recognition. One large retrospective survey
suggested that 40% of patients had complex seizures in the first
decade of life.

Attacks are often limited to distorted sensations and restricted
semi-purposive movements without secondary generalization
and tonic-clonic movements.

18.7   The following are recognized associations

A   sodium valproate and transient hair loss
B   sodium valproate and appetite suppression
C   carbamazepine and Stevens–Johnson syndrome
D   rectal diazepam and apnoea
E   phenytoin chewable tablets and dental caries

18.8   Febrile convulsions

A   occur in between 3 and 4% of children
B   have a peak incidence between 6 and 12 months
C   are usually brief, generalized tonic-clonic episodes
D   are more common in boys
E   are the major cause of partial complex seizures in later
      childhood

18.9   The following features are compatible with a syncopal attack

A   absence of deathly pallor
B   clonic movements
C   urinary incontinence
D   age under 2 years
E   bitten tongue

(Answers overleaf)

18.7 **A C D**
Anticonvulsants are associated with a formidable list of potential
side-effects; fortunately, most are rare but clinicians need to
consider the risks when deciding on long-term drug exposure.
Parents expect to be warned of side-effects and how they should
recognize them. It can be a formidable task to communicate not
only a diagnosis of epilepsy but also to provide a balanced view
of the cost–benefit ratio of anticonvulsants.

The commonly used anticonvulsants, valproate and
carbamazepine, have good safety profiles but reference should
be made to the published side-effects list, e.g. the *British
National Formulary*. Valproate may produce gastric irritation and
nausea, but in the longer term it increases appetite and weight
gain. Valproate may also cause transient hair loss.

Carbamazepine commonly produces a transient erythematous
skin rash but may also provoke a full-blown Stevens–Johnson
syndrome.

Rectal diazepam solution is a convenient formulation for
controlling prolonged seizures but the rapid absorption may
result in depressed respiration.

Anticonvulsants were in the past administered as sugar-
containing suspensions, and caries was prevalent in epileptic
children. Alternatives are now available. In the case of phenytoin
there is a specific problem of gum hypertrophy.

18.8 **A C D**
Febrile convulsions are rare below age 6 months, and after age
5 years; the peak age range is 9–20 months. Boys outnumber
girls, and show a different age-related pattern reflecting the sex
difference in brain maturation. Girls mature faster and show a
sharper decline in the incidence of febrile convulsions.

Most authorities now believe that children who are
neurologically normal have a very low risk of developing
epilepsy after one or more febrile convulsions. Fever may,
however, be the trigger which provokes prolonged, complex
febrile convulsions in young children already predisposed to
epileptic attacks.

18.9 **B C D E**
In spite of the characteristic features of innocent syncopal
attacks, readily confirmed by an adequate history, they are too
commonly confused with epilepsy. Warning sensations and a
deathly pallor inevitably precede a faint. The loss of
consciousness is a matter of seconds unless the child is held
upright, in which case it may be longer! The child may briefly
stiffen or have a few clonic movements; incontinence is possible
and the tongue can be damaged during the fall.

18.10 The following disorders would explain repeated sudden loss of consciousness in a 2-year-old child

A habit spasms
B breath-holding attacks
C reflex anoxic seizures
D benign paroxysmal vertigo
E masturbation

18.11 Duchenne muscular dystrophy

A affecting a boy indicates that his mother is an obligate carrier
B is consistently associated with an elevated plasma creatine kinase level
C should be suspected in a boy not walking by the age of 18 months
D should be suspected in a boy unable to run by age 2 years
E does not directly involve the central nervous system

18.12 Myotonic dystrophy

A is inherited as an X-linked condition
B is a cause of respiratory failure in the neonate
C is associated with intellectual delay
D is restricted to skeletal musculature
E causes frontal hair loss during childhood

18.13 The following features support the diagnosis of infectious polyneuritis (Guillain-Barré syndrome)

A involvement of both distal and proximal muscles
B asymmetrical limb weakness
C CSF pleocytosis
D mild bilateral facial weakness
E progression of weakness limited to a few days

(Answers overleaf)

18.10 **B C**
There are several potential causes of repeated impaired attention and abnormal movement but few options when it comes to explaining recurrent loss of consciousness in a child who is otherwise healthy.

Breath-holding attacks are usually apparent from the history of crying and becoming blue. Reflex anoxic seizures can be notoriously difficult to differentiate from epilepsy. There is not always a precipitating event to trigger the vagally-mediated bradycardia, and the pallor and floppyness may be accompanied by brief abnormal movements.

18.11 **B C D**
The X chromosome locus responsible for Duchenne muscular dystrophy is large and contains several alleles. It follows that the manifestations in affected boys are variable, and that biochemical markers in definite and probable carriers are inconsistent. The mutation rate is high, and may account for a third of newly recognized cases; the problem for family studies is whether the mutation has occurred in mother or son. There is rapidly growing experience in the application of gene probe procedures and, when refined, these should revolutionize family counselling and antenatal diagnosis.

Early recognition of affected boys is possible by measuring creatine kinase levels in late or unsteady walkers.

A proportion have mild to moderate mental handicap associated with abnormal EEGs and CT evidence of cortical atrophy.

18.12 **B C**
Myotonic dystrophy is inherited as an autosomal dominant with incomplete penetrance. Without careful family review it may not be evident that there is an inherited problem. You should at least shake the hands and watch the smiles of parents whose floppy infant is having breathing difficulties in your neonatal unit!

Progressive mental handicap is a feature, particularly in those with early onset weakness. Myocardial involvement is common, as are other systemic manifestations. However, frontal baldness and cataracts are limited to adults.

18.13 **A D E**
It is vital not to overlook a lesion causing spinal cord compression. Warning signs would include asymmetrical weakness, disproportionate sphincter disturbance and a detectable level below which there is neurological impairment. Permitted CSF findings include a normal or borderline cell count increase and a marked elevation of protein level.

18.14 The following are early signs of raised intracranial pressure in infancy

A   papilloedema
B   cracked-pot sound
C   bulging fontanelle
D   cranial bruit
E   skull X-ray abnormalities

18.15 A cerebellar astrocytoma is suggested by

A   a fixed head tilt
B   early morning vomiting
C   grand mal attacks
D   cranial diabetes insipidus
E   slowly progressive facial weakness

18.16 Migraine

A   is rare in pre-school children
B   is suggested when vomiting starts after the onset of headache
C   is unlikely if headache is bilateral
D   is associated with susceptibility to travel sickness
E   may be accompanied by an abnormal EEG

18.17 Cerebral palsy

A   is the commonest cause of severe physical disability in children
B   has become less common over the last decade as obstetric practice has improved
C   has a clear-cut relationship to perinatal factors in less than 10% of cases
D   is associated with a greater than 20% death rate before age 20 years
E   is increasing in prevalence in very low birthweight infants

(Answers overleaf)

18.14 **C**
   Palpation of the fontanelle and sutures, together with careful
   attention to skull circumference measurements, is the most
   reliable sign. Papilloedema, and a cracked-pot sound on skull
   percussion, applies to older children with closed sutures. The
   absence of papilloedema does not exclude raised intracranial
   pressure.

18.15 **A B**
   Infratentorial tumours predominate in the 2–15 year age group.
   Cerebellar astrocytomas are slow growing and often cystic.
   They manifest themselves through ataxia and gradually
   increasing intracranial pressure. A fixed head tilt, the direction of
   tilt being constant, may be an early sign. The child is usually
   unaware of tilt. Early diagnosis provides for an excellent
   outcome in the majority of cases.

18.16 **B D E**
   The story of migraine is complete normality between
   headaches. A positive family history and characteristic
   progression from prodromal symptoms to headache to nausea
   and vomiting provide confirmation but the pattern in young
   children may be atypical. Migraine is reported to increase in
   frequency with age but this is partly due to under-recognition in
   the pre-school age group. Younger children are unable to
   describe the aura phase and tend to have bilateral rather than
   unilateral headaches. The headache usually ceases with the
   onset of nausea and vomiting. If vomiting consistently precedes
   headache, investigations are required to exclude cerebral
   tumour, partial epilepsy, and metabolic errors
   (hyperammonaemia, lactic acidosis).
       EEGs in migraine may show mild wave abnormalities.

18.17 **A C E**
   Cerebral palsy is a symptom complex rather than a single entity,
   and data on incidence and prevalence are inexact. Estimates
   vary between 2 and 4 cases per 1000 births, and there is no
   evidence of a recent decline despite improved obstetric
   standards. This is understandable when it is recognized that
   cerebral palsy has a stronger correlation with adverse factors in
   pregnancy rather than in labour. Birth asphyxia is hard to define
   and measure but studies suggest that perinatal factors account
   for approximately 8% of cerebral palsy. This statistic obviously
   has important implications when resolving legal claims.
       Recent studies have shown that the survival of children with
   mild to moderate cerebral palsy differs little from normal children.
   Amongst the most disabled group survival is still around 50%.
   The life expectancy of children with cerebral palsy has important
   implications for social, educational and health services.

18.18 Spastic hemiparesis

   A   usually results in greater disability of leg rather than arm
   B   does not delay walking in the majority of cases
   C   results in asymmetrical growth failure
   D   is commonly associated with epilepsy
   E   does not result in impaired sensation

18.19 The following are recognized causes of cerebral palsy

   A   hypoxic-ischaemic encephalopathy
   B   ataxia telangiectasis
   C   spinal cord tumour
   D   non-accidental injury
   E   familial spastic paraparesis

18.20 Meningitis is a recognized cause of the following complications

   A   hyponatraemia
   B   gastrointestinal haemorrhage
   C   sensorineural deafness
   D   optic atrophy
   E   periventricular leukomalacia

(Answers overleaf)

18.18 **B C D**
The arm is typically more involved, and initial recognition often follows the observation that early hand manipulation is asymmetrical. In general, hemiparetic children do not have delayed walking. Depending on severity there is restricted growth of the involved limbs. This can lead to marked differences in hand and foot size, or be as subtle as a discrepancy in nail size. Disturbances in sensation are present but may be difficult to define objectively. They particularly affect body image.

18.19 **A D**
The term 'cerebral palsy' is convenient shorthand for describing a disorder of posture and movement due to a static lesion of the developing brain. The diagnostic danger is that progressive disorders may mimic the early dynamic stage of cerebral palsy. The correct diagnosis may dramatically alter the management and prognosis of the child, and may have genetic implications.

The pregnancy and birth history may reveal a clear explanation for presumed cerebral palsy, but cerebral imaging with ultrasound, CT or MRI is always justified. Ataxic cerebral palsy is probably the form most likely to be confused with a progressive disorder such as ataxia telangiectasia or certain metabolic errors, e.g. metachromatic leukodystrophy or hexosaminidase A and B deficiency.

18.20 **A B C D**
Meningitis may be followed by a range of early and late complications. Pneumococcal meningitis is the potentially most damaging of the bacterial causes in childhood but neonatal meningitis also carries a high morbidity. Meningitis is often associated with septicaemia and hence the hazards of shock and disseminated intravascular coagulation. Inappropriate secretion of antidiuretic hormone has to be anticipated and hyponatraemia avoided by fluid restriction and attention to plasma electrolyte values.

Deafness is described in as many as 10% of patients after bacterial meningitis. Recent trials have suggested that dexamethasone administration immediately prior to commencement of antibiotics reduces later hearing deficit. The penalty may be an increased risk of stress ulceration and gastric haemorrhage.

19. Vision, hearing, speech

19.1 A squint

A does not require formal evaluation until it has persisted beyond age 6 months

B may be within normal up to age 18 months if transient and unilateral

C is more frequent in children with epicanthic folds

D is more frequently due to hypermetropia than myopia

E in a young child is more likely to be divergent rather than convergent

19.2 The following statements about visual development are correct

A the red reflex is absent before 36 weeks gestation

B newborn infants follow slowly moving objects

C the visual acuity of newborn infants is better than 6/24

D a visual acuity of 6/6 should be achieved by age 4 years

E random, unco-ordinated eye movements should not be present after age 6 weeks

19.3 Cataracts are a recognized feature of

A extreme prematurity

B congenital rubella

C galactosaemia

D Tay–Sach disease

E fetal alcohol syndrome

19.4 The following signs are useful guides to intact hearing in an infant

A a newborn infant should open his eyes widely in response to a sudden loud noise

B at age 1 month he should turn to a prolonged sound

C at age 3 months he should quieten or smile to the sound of his mother's voice

D at age 4–5 months he should successfully perform a distraction test

E at age 9 months he should show pleasure in babbling loudly and tunefully

(Answers overleaf)

19.1   **B D**
Occasional and unsustained ocular deviation is common in infants of less than 6 months of age. Transient squints of only a few seconds duration may be acceptable up to 18 months. However, more marked or constant squints should not be accepted as physiological at any age. Hypermetropia is a common cause of the more prevalent convergent squint. Myopia can present with ocular deviation, more usually the less frequent divergent concomitant strabismus.

19.2   **B D E**
It is important to have a general understanding of visual development. More than 70% of early learning is dependent on vision. Unfortunately vision screening remains one of the more inadequate components of child health surveillance, and vision testing of young children is notoriously difficult even in experienced hands.

Eliciting the red reflex is a basic procedure for establishing that the gross anatomy of the eye is intact. An absent red reflex in a newborn, even if premature, raises the suspicion of congenital abnormality.

Babies will fix on clearly contrasting objects from 33 weeks gestation. Newborn term infants will fix and follow objects which are moved slowly in the horizontal plane. Vertical tracking emerges from age 4–8 weeks. Visual acuity approximates to 6/200 at birth, improving to 6/60 by 3 months and 6/12 by 2–3 years. A school entry child should be able to co-operate with acuity testing using a linear (Snellen) chart at 6 metres.

A baby who has nystagmus or wobbly eye movements requires specialist evaluation of potential visual or neurological disorders.

19.3   **B C**
Congenital rubella, toxoplasmosis, cytomegalovirus and Herpes simplex infection cause cataracts. Systemic causes include galactosaemia, galactokinase deficiency, hypoparathyroidism, Lowe syndrome and mannosidosis. They may be inherited as an autosomal dominant, and 50% are of sporadic unknown aetiology.

19.4   **A C E**
Parental observation is a valuable aspect of health screening and this is especially true in the detection of deafness. Many health authorities distribute checklists incorporating hints for parents; the correct items listed in the question are derived from the list prepared by Dr Barry McCormick. Failure to achieve items on the list will alert the Health Visitor to arrange formal assessment either with a distraction test between 7 and 9 months, or by referral to a specialist hearing assessment unit.

19.5 The following have a recognized association with deafness
    A cleft palate
    B head injury
    C retinitis pigmentosa
    D congenital cytomegalovirus infection
    E bacterial meningitis

19.6 Late speech may be caused by
    A stammering
    B fragile X syndrome
    C autism
    D elective mutism
    E congenital rubella

(Answers overleaf)

19.5   **A B C D E**
Significant conductive hearing loss will be found in 5–10% of children at some time. The majority results from secretory otitis media. Children with congenital structural problems of the upper airway such as cleft or high-arched palates are especially vulnerable.

Sensorineural deafness occurs in 3 per 1000 children and up to 50% have a genetic basis. It is therefore important to check the family history and to look for other components of potential syndromes. Retinitis pigmentosa and deafness are linked in Usher syndrome, an autosomal recessive disorder.

19.6   **B C E**
Stammering is common in preschool children and is usually no more than a lack of fluency at the stage of rapid expansion of vocabulary and increase in sentence length. In a minority, stammering becomes persistent and interferes in language progression and social interaction. It is not a cause of late speech.

Fragile X syndrome is an example of a disorder in which general delay may first manifest as language problems.

Language disorder is a characteristic presentation of autism. Acquired loss of speech may also be due to acquired deafness, neurodegenerative disease or rare patterns of epilepsy. Elective mutism is usually apparent when a child has normal language in the home but not in school or other social settings.

Congenital rubella and cytomegalovirus may result in not only sensorineural deafness but also coexistent cognitive defects.

20. Mental handicap

20.1 Severe learning difficulty has a recognized association with
- **A** fetal alcohol syndrome
- **B** juvenile hypothyroidism
- **C** Turner syndrome
- **D** Tuberose sclerosis
- **E** fragile X syndrome

20.2 Severe learning difficulty
- **A** has no recognized cause in the majority of affected children
- **B** is more prevalent in children of manual and unemployed parents
- **C** is more frequent in males
- **D** has a recognized association with epilepsy
- **E** is commonly linked to behavioural problems

20.3 Children with moderate learning difficulty
- **A** frequently have siblings with similar problems
- **B** often have a normal measured IQ
- **C** have often been exposed to complicated births
- **D** are more at risk from abuse
- **E** are more at risk from cigarette smoke

(Answers overleaf)

20.1 **A D E**
Developmental delay and neurological dysfunction are the most sensitive indicators of maternal alcohol consumption in pregnancy. The behavioural, intellectual and motor defects can occur without suggestive craniofacial malformation but there tends to be a parallel with growth failure.

Juvenile or acquired hypothyroidism may reduce school performance but it rarely leads to severe, irreversible intellectual problems; this is a marked contrast with late-treated congenital hypothyroidism.

It is a common misconception that girls with Turner syndrome have severely reduced intelligence. Their intelligence distribution, particularly for linguistic skills, is close to the normal population. It is only in tests related to spatial and abstract concepts that they score poorly.

20.2 **C D E**
The term severe learning difficulty is replacing mental handicap, and emphasizes that the education process has to be adjusted to accommodate these children. Severe learning difficulties occur in approximately 3.5 per 1000 population. The majority have a recognized cause, most frequently a chromosomal or central nervous system abnormality, and parents and siblings are usually of normal ability. There is an excess of males partly due to sex-linked recessively inherited conditions, such as fragile X syndrome.

A high proportion of people with severe learning difficulties develop epilepsy, either during childhood or in early adult life. Challenging behaviour is also a common problem and adds to the multiplicity of handicaps facing these children and their families.

20.3 **A B D E**
Moderate learning difficulty is as much a marker of socio-economic deprivation as it is of below average ability. Children classified as having moderate learning difficulty are likely to have parents who are categorized as manual or unemployed. Family size is above average with resultant overcrowding, as well as increased exposure to damp and cigarette smoke. Brothers and sisters often repeat the pattern of deprivation and poor school performance. There is also an association with physical and sexual abuse as well as neglect. It is important for the educational and health care teams to recognize these issues and provide a comprehensive and easily accessible support network.

20.4 Clinical features characteristically associated with identifiable causes of mental handicap include
A corneal clouding
B a sweet odour
C bluish pigmentation over the lower back
D genu valgum
E broad thumbs

20.5 Phenylketonuria
A results from failure of phenylalanine conversion to phenylpyruvate
B may be reliably screened for on the basis of blood analysis at age 48 hours
C screening allows over half of affected children to complete normal schooling
D requires dietary control throughout childhood
E results in reduction of neurotransmitter amine synthesis

20.6 Tay–Sach disease
A is amenable to prevention by population screening for heterozygote status
B results in a depressed startle response to sound
C causes motor weakness beginning between 3 and 6 months
D causes microcephaly
E is associated with red spot in the macular region of the retina

20.7 Gaucher disease
A is, in its usual form, primarily a disease of the central nervous system
B results from deficiency of the enzyme that cleaves glucose from ceramide
C results from lipid accumulation within the cells of the reticuloendothelial system
D is a cause of episodic bone pain
E is a cause of chronic thrombocytopenia

(Answers overleaf)

20.4   **A B E**
Detailed examination and obsessionally careful documentation
is an essential part of reviewing the infant or child with delayed
development. This may reveal a pattern of dysmorphic features
which enables appropriate investigation and diagnosis. In these
examples corneal clouding, a coarsened facies and
hepatosplenomegaly, would have led to the recognition of
mucopolysaccharidosis. Smelling sick infants may put you on
the track of metabolic errors, e.g. maple syrup urine disease.
Hand examination is a good introduction to any patient! Broad
thumbs and big toes, together with short stature, downward
slanting palpebral fissures and hypoplastic maxilla match the
description of Rubinstein–Taybi syndrome.

20.5   **C D E**
Phenylketonuria, or hyperphenylalaninaemia, results from
deficiency of phenylalanine hydroxylase (or its cofactor), the
enzyme responsible for converting phenylalanine to tyrosine.
The resulting urinary metabolites are too inconsistent and
unstable to allow reliable detection. Blood phenylalanine
measurement is reliable as long as the sample is taken with the
baby established on milk feeding.
    The outcome of early treated patients appears good in that
average IQs are at, or just below, the standardized population
mean of 100. However, the mean IQ remains below that of
unaffected siblings, and behavioural and psychometric problems
reduce overall school performance. Performance falls further
when diet is relaxed and plasma phenylalanine levels rise. The
current approach is to attempt to maintain some dietary control
for as long as possible.

20.6   **A C E**
Tay–Sach disease is the commonest ganglioside storage disease,
and has been linked to a mutation on chromosome 15 causing
hexosaminidase A deficiency. The heterozygote frequency among
Ashkenazi Jewish people is 1 in 27. Heterozygotes can be reliably
detected by serum assay. A highly motivated population together
with antenatal diagnosis has made this the first condition to be
prevented by mass screening of at-risk populations.
    An exaggerated startle response to sudden noise is a
characteristic early sign. The neuronal lipidosis results in
macrocephaly.

20.7   **B C D E**
Type 1 or chronic non-neuropathic Gaucher disease accounts
for a large majority of this disorder. The usual features are
hepatosplenomegaly, hypersplenism and bone lesions. The
natural history is variable but central nervous involvement is
uncommon. Types 2 and 3 are neuronopathic forms, and the
patterns appear to be genetically distinct.

20.8 Features of mucopolysaccharide storage disease include
   A abnormally shaped vertebral bodies
   B stiff joints
   C cataracts
   D coronary artery obstruction
   E distinctive aminoaciduria

(Answer overleaf)

20.8   **A B D**
With some exceptions, the mucopolysaccharidoses share
several characteristic features, notably short stature and skeletal
deformity, stiff joints, corneal clouding, deafness, abnormal
arterial wall deposits, hepatosplenomegaly and progressive
intellectual deterioration. Diagnosis is confirmed by measuring
urinary dermatan and heparan sulphate, followed by studying
specific lysosomal enzymes.

21. Behaviour

21.1 Clumsy children

    A make up 5–15% of the school population
    B are largely accounted for by the effects of mild to moderate birth asphyxia
    C are frequently slow to develop laterality
    D usually demonstrate abnormally increased limb tone
    E tend to have delayed speech

21.2 Specific reading retardation

    A affects approximately 5% of primary school children
    B is primarily due to delayed visual word perception (word blindness)
    C is associated with erratic eye movement during reading
    D is more prevalent among boys
    E is usually compensated for by above average achievement in arithmetic

21.3 Nocturnal enuresis

    A occurs in approximately 5% of 5 year olds
    B has an organic basis in around 2%
    C persisting until age 8 years is an indication for renal ultrasound measurement
    D is commoner in social classes IV and V
    E is associated with sleeplessness

21.4 Faecal soiling

    A is abnormal if it occurs in a 5 year old
    B is often associated with constipation
    C may be due to lax training procedures
    D is caused by an abnormality of the rectum in about 10% of affected children
    E is an indication for a low roughage diet

(Answers overleaf)

21.1 **A C E**
This is a common problem in which children show difficulty in
motor co-ordination out of proportion to their general ability.
Few have objective evidence of birth asphyxia, and it is better to
regard it as part of a normal spectrum. It is probable that it
reflects both genetic and environmental factors. Hypotonia,
delayed laterality, and poor mouth co-ordination are all features,
and they can lead to secondary problems of loss of confidence
and social isolation.

21.2 **A C D**
Among children of average intelligence who experience
difficulties in learning to read, write and spell, the majority have
a basic defect of language development. A minority, around
10%, have a disturbance of visual perception. Word blindness is
therefore an inappropriate term for the whole condition. Normal
readers move their eyes in an orderly fashion from left to right
across the page. These children show more erratic movements,
and more movements from right to left. Arithmetic also suffers
because of sequencing problems, and because of general loss
of confidence.

21.3 **B D**
At age 5 years, 15% or 1 in 8 wet their bed; by 10 years the
figure is down to around 5% and by 15 years, 1%. Urinary
infection is more common in children with nocturnal enuresis,
but routine urinary tract investigation cannot be justified without
additional evidence, notably positive urine cultures. Children
with this problem tend to be deep sleepers. They even manage
to sleep through the din created by enuresis alarms, when the
rest of the household has been awakened!

21.4 **A B C**
Any child starting school at 5 years of age and still soiling his
trousers has a problem that justifies further enquiry. Many will
be found to have associated constipation and the soiling is due
to soft stools passing around the impacted faecal masses. In
others it may be a matter of failure of training. After these two
common underlying factors have been excluded, more serious
behaviour disturbances must be considered. It is very unlikely,
however, that even in this selected group structural rectal
abnormalities will be found.

21.5 Tics

A are repetitive purposeful movements
B are rare in the preschool child
C occur in 4–5% of children
D are commonly familial
E commonly persist into adult life

21.6 Features of autism include

A onset of behaviour disturbance before age 30 months
B delay in speech and language development
C frequent association of partial seizures
D echolalia
E sensorineural deafness

21.7 Presentations highly suggestive of non-accidental injury include

A seizures and retinal haemorrhages in a 3 month old
B greenstick fracture of the tibia in a 3 year old
C bruised fingertips in a 20 month old
D palatal and gum bruising in a 6 month old
E a single anal fissure and perianal erythema in a 2 year old

21.8 Sexual abuse

A is more likely to be perpetrated by a relative than a non-relative
B accounts for less than 10% of all cases of abuse
C involves girls rather than boys with a ratio of around 20 to 1
D involves children aged under 5 years in approximately a third of cases
E is associated with confirmatory physical signs in about 80% of cases

(Answers overleaf)

21.5 **C D**
Tics are surprisingly common and commence as early as age 2
years. Only when they are severe, persistent and a disturbance,
is the child likely to be taken to a doctor. The movements
usually have no purpose and are most common in the face and
neck. In as many as 25% there is a family history. Tics usually
disappear, often in late adolescence.

21.6 **A B D**
The four diagnostic criteria described by Rutter include early
failure to exhibit interpersonal relationships, delay in language
development, ritualistic and compulsive phenomena, and onset
before age 30 months.

21.7 **A D**
The identification of an abused child is based on a
comprehensive assessment of the child and his family. The
paediatrician must be familiar with the range of injuries that may
arise by accident, and alert to those that do not match the
presenting history.
    Anal pathology may cause you to consider the possibility of
sexual abuse. A single fissure and erythema in themselves are
not highly suggestive.

21.8 **A D**
It can be argued that we are still ignorant of the true
epidemiology of childhood sexual abuse. In the UK, recognized
cases are increasing exponentially. Sexual abuse accounted for
over 30% of children placed on NSPCC 'at risk' registers in 1986.
The sex ratio of abused children is nearer 2.5 girls to 1 boy. Anal
abuse is common in boys of all ages and in young girls. Vaginal
abuse becomes more prevalent after age 6–8 years.
    An examination where no abnormality is found cannot
exclude abuse. Surveys of abused girls have shown no
confirmatory findings in around 70%.

Case histories

CASE 1 UNEXPECTED DEATH
A week-old child is found dead in her cot when her mother goes to feed her at 8.00 am. The infant was born normally, birthweight 3.5 kg, was the first child and had fed reasonably well. It would be appropriate to advise the parents that

A   a post-mortem is unlikely to reveal any pathology
B   there is no risk of a similar tragedy affecting any further children they may have
C   it is advisable to delay having further children for a year or so
D   that the child's mother should seek professional advice if she is still grieving in 3 months
E   that she may have problems carrying the next infant to term

CASE 2 AN UNEXPECTED FINDING
Whilst examining a boy aged 10 years, who presents with a chest infection, you hear an ejection systolic murmur at the left sternal edge which is not transmitted up into the neck. The heart sounds are normal, and there are no other added sounds. The heart rate and rhythm as assessed from the radial pulse are normal. You should

A   tell the child and parents of your finding
B   arrange for an ECG
C   arrange for an echocardiogram
D   provide advice on antibiotic prophylaxis before dental procedures
E   refer to a cardiologist

(Answers overleaf)

CASE 1   C

Sudden death within a week of birth is far more likely to be due to a known disorder, particularly heart abnormalities, and therefore careful and detailed post-mortems are essential. Congenital heart defects are polygenically inherited and there is a higher risk on future pregnancies, but it is usually small. Metabolic disorders are usually recessively inherited and there is therefore a 1 in 4 risk with all future pregnancies.

To help the parents, particularly the mother, to recover from the pregnancy and loss of their baby, it is prudent to delay planning further children for a year or so, and not to try and immediately replace the one they have lost. Sadness at the loss lasts longer than most people think and is often at its worst 3 months after the event. This is to be anticipated and it helps if they are warned about it. Excessive grieving always requires professional support.

CASE 2   **None**

An ejection systolic murmur at the left sternal edge is a common finding which may be of no clinical significance. It is essential to examine the child thoroughly for any other evidence of a heart disorder; this includes clinical assessment of heart size and ventricular activity, blood pressure and pulses in lower limbs. If all is normal it is appropriate to check him again at a later opportunity when he has recovered from the chest infection. If the murmur persists but is not of any functional significance the boy and his parents can be told that he, like many others, has an innocent murmur.

CASE 3 UNUSUAL INHERITANCE

A 20-year-old mother, who is stunted due to severe bowing of the legs despite large doses of vitamin D, calcium and phosphate supplementation to her diet during most of her childhood, brings her 2-month-old baby daughter to clinic seeking advice. Her baby weighed 4 kg at birth and is breastfeeding and growing well. It would be correct to tell her

A   that rickets resistant to treatment with large doses of vitamins is a sex-linked disorder

B   that girls are as likely to be affected as boys

C   that the basic defect is due to loss of phosphate rather than lack of vitamin D

D   that breast milk is poor in vitamin D and therefore she should change to artificial feeding

E   that in view of her child's good birthweight and early growth she is unlikely to be suffering from the same disorder

CASE 4 A CONFIDENT DIAGNOSIS

A baby is born in the early hours of the morning by spontaneous vertex delivery at 38 weeks gestation and weighed 3.1 kg. At 09.00 hours his mother puts him to the breast but he does not suckle. She asks the midwife for help. The midwife wonders if the child has Down syndrome and calls you to do an 'early' routine examination. You record the following abnormal features in the notes: an apparent squint, a 3rd fontanelle, white spots in the periphery of the iris, a single palmar crease on the right hand, generalized hypotonia and hyperextensibility. You also note that the pulses and heart sounds are normal and there are no murmurs.

A   you would be correct to tell the midwife that all the positive signs you have recorded are more common in infants with Down syndrome

B   you would be right to conclude that there was no significant heart defect present

C   you would not speak to his parents until you had the results of chromosome studies

D   you would arrange for an X-ray of the neck

E   the reluctance of the infant to feed is one of the first signs of duodenal atresia

(Answers overleaf)

CASE 3   **A   B   C**

Vitamin D-resistant rickets or familial hypophosphataemic rickets is inherited as a sex-linked dominant disorder. Most sex-linked disorders are recessive, which means that mothers are carriers and 50% of sons are affected. In sex-linked dominant disorders 50% of *sons and daughters* are affected. Breast milk is low in vitamin D but that is not a reason to abandon breast milk feeding in this child or any other. Vitamin D supplements can be given if required.

   A defect in renal phosphate reabsorption is accepted as the primary lesion in familial hypophosphataemic rickets. Affected children do not manifest the rickets and deformity before the end of the first year of life. Low plasma phosphate and increased alkaline phosphatase levels, judged against age-related standards, provide for early diagnosis.

CASE 4   **A**

It is often possible to be confident about the diagnosis of Down syndrome on the clinical features alone. It is the picture as a whole which is convincing and not any one individual feature. None of those which you recorded is of itself diagnostic.

   Heart defects may not be detected by clinical examination alone. All infants with Down syndrome require imaging to fully exclude a heart defect.

   Under usual circumstances you should not examine a child without first seeking the parents' permission. There is no excuse for not doing so in this instance. You therefore must go back and tell the parents what you found and what you recommend. You need not share all your anxieties with them, so if they do not ask, you may elect not to mention Down syndrome if you are not confident of the diagnosis on the basis of your clinical examination.

   Children with Down syndrome do have problems with the stability of the first two cervical vertebrae, but an X-ray at this time is not indicated. Infants with isolated duodenal atresia suck well enough.

CASE 5 FETAL ALCOHOL SYNDROME

A woman married to a man of importance finds she is 4 months pregnant. Her lifestyle includes social dinners and cocktail parties. She says she drinks fewer than two or three gin and tonics each day. She comes to you seeking reassurance. It would be correct to say

A   that two or three gin and tonics with food is unlikely to have caused any harm

B   that the majority of children born to known alcoholic mothers show no sign of damage at birth or in their development over their early years

C   that abstinence for the remainder of the pregnancy is unlikely to reduce the risk of damage very much

D   that affected infants are easily recognized at birth by their characteristic facial appearance

E   that if the infant is small but appears otherwise normal then he is unlikely to have come to any harm

CASE 6 BIRTH ASPHYXIA

A 4.2 kg newborn infant was born head first by forceps delivery because of maternal distress, delay in 2nd stage, and fetal tachycardia. The mother required heavy sedation. The infant gasped at birth but did not begin regular breathing immediately, the pharyngeal aspirate contained meconium and vernix, the heart rate at birth was around 160 and remained high. At 1 minute the infant made another gasp and by 4 minutes regular respiration had commenced and the infant became pink. The infant's subsequent progress was uneventful. Unfortunately the child has cerebral palsy. The parents wish to know why. It would be correct to say

A   there is evidence that this baby was asphyxiated before birth

B   there is no evidence that the child's brain was damaged by that asphyxia

C   there is no evidence that the child was damaged by the forceps

D   the child's good postnatal progress excludes a prenatal cause of brain damage

E   only rarely does birth asphyxia result in cerebral palsy

(Answers overleaf)

CASE 5   **B   C**

This is not an easy question. It feels comfortable to reassure worried parents but not at the cost of misleading them. There is epidemiological evidence that two to three gin and tonics (which she admits to) can cause damage, but on the other hand a majority of infants born to known alcoholics appear unaffected. The damage, in the main, appears to occur in the early months of gestation — dysmorphism, associated heart and renal defects. Obviously abstinence could only benefit the infant. The facial abnormalities are subtle and not easily recognized. The 'fetal alcohol syndrome' is defined by facial features, intrauterine growth retardation, neurodevelopmental abnormalities and a variety of congenital abnormalities. The term 'fetal alcohol effects' has been coined for the lesser effects, low birthweight with learning and behaviour problems would be an example.

CASE 6   **A   B   C   E**

Fetal tachycardia, meconium aspiration and delayed onset of respiration are features of fetal asphyxia. They may occur in a fetus distressed for whatever reason. The infant's heart rate was good at birth, and his subsequent progress was uneventful. There is therefore no evidence of a brain damaging event at the time of birth, and no grounds for confirming either asphyxia or trauma as the cause of brain damage. It has to be emphasized that a baby with an ill-formed brain, or one damaged in early pregnancy may give no sign of it in early life. In many instances the aetiology of cerebral palsy is not known. It is a mistake to ascribe it to perinatal asphyxia in the absence of signs of brain damage in the immediate newborn period.

CASE 7 A WELL-INFORMED PARENT
An insulin-dependent diabetic mother was delivered of a female
infant at 33 weeks gestation who weighed 3.3 kg. The infant became
breathless and required extra oxygen. Despite suckling at the breast,
the infant's blood sugar became unmeasurable and intravenous
glucose was required for 48 hours. Jaundice developed and
phototherapy was given. At 3 weeks all was well and the infant went
home. The mother is knowledgeable about diabetes. She has some
questions for you. Would it be correct to tell her that

A   her baby was overweight and that it was a consequence of her
     diabetes
B   that the blood glucose would not have dropped if the infant had
     been able to take more feed
C   jaundice is more common in infants born of diabetic mothers
D   that no event occurred after birth which might be expected to
     compromise her child's future
E   that in contrast to her 'Islets of Langerhan' which were under
     performing, her infant's Islet cells would be hypertrophied and over
     performing

CASE 8 A CYANOSED BABY
The midwife on the lying-in ward is concerned because a term infant
became cyanosed and breathless whilst feeding and has remained
so. It would be appropriate to

A   give a test feed
B   check the apex beat
C   pass a tube into the stomach
D   pass a tube into the rectum
E   take blood cultures and give penicillin

(Answers overleaf)

CASE 7 A C E

It is always a challenge to know what to say to parents who have read the books and may be as well informed as you are. Unlike you, they are also the parents of the child and subject to real and imagined anxieties about their child's welfare and future. So they need to be told the truth, but not necessarily all you know, with the attendant uncertainties. *White lies* in the best interest of the child should be used sparingly.

So, yes the child was overweight, and yes it was due to her diabetic state. But no, the blood sugar falls despite the most successful feeding programmes, even though the intravenous glucose is not always required. Yes, jaundice is more common but it is not a serious problem. It is (D) which is the testing question. The infant cannot be the better for being born too early, developing hypoglycaemia and becoming jaundiced. So, to say nothing with potential deleterious sequelae happened would be incorrect, but it would be wrong to emphasize the risks, or to dwell on the epidemiological data unless pressed.

CASE 8 B C D E

It is essential to ensure that certain conditions are excluded which can be life threatening if overlooked. They include oesophageal atresia, usually associated with a tracheo-oesophageal fistula (and occasionally with rectal atresia), and diaphragmatic hernia. The association with a feed may be fortuitous; a feed 'exercises' the infant. Infection and in particular Group B streptococcal infection should be suspected in all such situations and systemic penicillin given until diagnosis can be discounted.

CASE 9 A BLEEDING INFANT
A 5-day-old breastfed infant begins to bleed from her gums and umbilical stump, and blood is found in the stool. On examination she has a fluctuating erythematous rash, blue–black patches of size 5–10 cm across over the base of the back and buttocks, and dark salmon marks 1–2 cm diameter on the nape of the neck. It would be good practice to

A tell her parents that the erythematous rash is usually of no importance and will soon disappear
B tell her parents that the pigmented patches are called 'Mongolian blue spots' and they have no medical significance
C say that salmon patches are found in over 30% of infants and are not associated with abnormalities elsewhere
D enquire if she had been given vitamin K, and if not, give her an intramuscular therapeutic dose
E recommend that the breast milk be supplemented with an artifical feed

CASE 10 A LARGE INFANT
A slight, carefully dressed, young mother brings her large boisterous 1 year old to the outpatient department because her mother, mother-in-law and Health Visitor say he is too fat. Her husband is well built but not obese. On examination the infant is on the 90th percentile for length and above the 97th percentile for weight. She claims she can never satisfy his appetite. You should

A congratulate her for rearing a happy baby
B suggest she gives small frequent meals
C provide a 1000 Kcal diet sheet
D warn her that he is likely to remain obese
E perform skull X-rays with pituitary fossa views

CASE 11 MEASLES, MUMPS AND RUBELLA
A local parents' group has asked you to speak to them on the benefits of the combined measles, mumps and rubella vaccine. It would be correct to tell them

A measles can cause brain damage and death
B measles is particularly dangerous to children being treated for cancer
C mumps can cause deafness
D mumps is an important cause of sterility in females as well as males
E vaccinating boys against rubella is only justified on the basis of creating herd immunity

(Answers overleaf)

CASE 9 **A   C**

You may well disapprove of the answers, and consider the questions to be unhelpfully deceptive. 'Mongolian blue spots' is a widely used medical term, but it is not a helpful designation and may trigger unhelpful associations in the minds of parents. It is preferable to omit this name, and it might be helpful to explain that pigmented patches at the base of the spine are more common in peoples with dark skin.

Of course it would be proper to enquire if the child had been given vitamin K, but as the cause of this child's bleeding should be' presumed to be due to vitamin K deficiency, the child should be given a dose of vitamin K whether or not she had received vitamin K on the day of birth. Blood samples should be taken for investigations, including prothrombin level, before the vitamin K is administered.

CASE 10 **A   B**

In recent years we have possibly been too concerned about healthy young children who are a little overweight. It is, therefore, very appropriate to reassure this young mother threatened by knowning relatives and health advisers. It is said that obesity is less likely if the calories are given in small frequent amounts. Stricter dietary measures are inappropriate, though over indulgence and bad dietary habits should be avoided. It would be incorrect to state that he will inevitably become obese when he grows up although there is an association between obesity in childhood and in adults.

CASE 11 **A   B   C   E**

Complications of measles are rare but do include encephalitis and death. Children who are immunosuppressed as a result of being treated for cancer are particularly at risk of serious illness. Mumps is an important cause of deafness, but there is little evidence that it causes sterility in males or females. This is a common mis-understanding. It does cause painful orchitis. The ethical issue of giving boys a live vaccine to protect others has to be faced, but it could equally be argued that giving it to girls is to protect 'others' also.

CASE 12 TEMPERATURE STRIPS
A 3-week-old infant goes off his feed and becomes irritable. His teenage mother uses a 'temperature strip' on his forehead and is frightened to see it record 39°C. She arrives very distraught at the A&E department at 21.00 hours. When you approach the infant he appears to be peacefully asleep and his axillary temperature is 36.5°C. You should advise her that

A   in clinical practice, an infant's temperature can only be accurately recorded from the rectum
B   strips placed on the forehead can be inaccurate and cannot be relied upon
C   he needs to be admitted for observation
D   he should be given an antipyretic
E   it is vital to perform a lumbar puncture to exclude meningitis

CASE 13 'SUNDAY MORNING SYNDROME'
Parents drinking late on a Saturday night went to bed leaving bottles easily accessible. The following morning whilst the parents slept off the excess, their toddler found the bottles and drank the contents. He is brought to hospital 2 hours later, severely intoxicated. He is likely to suffer

A   hepatic necrosis
B   respiratory failure
C   severe metabolic acidosis
D   hypoglycaemia
E   profuse diarrhoea

CASE 14 A COMMON PROBLEM
A 4-year-old boy living with his grandparents has had four respiratory infections, each with a persistent cough, in the last 6 months. His grandma would be right when she says it might be due to

A   the bad weather this winter
B   his grandpa smoking like a chimney
C   a weak chest, just like his father, who suffered from bronchitis until he went into the army
D   him having no friends and always being in the house
E   him having his heart on the wrong side

(Answers overleaf)

CASE 12 **B C**

Parents recognize that a fever is a sign of illness. They usually measure the temperature to confirm what they already suspect. It is a matter of dispute as to how the temperature might be recorded accurately in infants. It is our view that it can be measured accurately from the axilla and that inserting instruments in the rectum is undesirable if it is unnecessary. Some temperature strips are inaccurate, but others are not. Recording the temperature from the forehead can give misleading results because the result is more influenced by the surroundings.

A 3-week-old infant who is reported to be 'off his feed', irritable and to have a fever, needs to be observed. A lumbar puncture is an intrusive test and should only be performed if indicated after fuller examination or further observation.

CASE 13 **B D**

The most serious consequence of acute alcohol intoxication in toddlers is brain damage due to hypoglycaemia.

CASE 14 **B C E**

This is a common complaint and there are few simple answers. Grandmas are formidable adversaries; only take them on when you are well armed and well protected. There is no point in disagreeing unless you have a convincing case. You could try telling her that 4 infections in the winter months, at 4 years of age, is about average. But statistics such as between 2 and 12, with an average of 6, attacks a year are cold comfort to anxious relatives. The incidence is higher in winter but attack rates do not correlate well with the weather. Smoking, either active or passive, is bad for everybody. An asthmatic tendency may be why he coughs with each infection. Mixing with children at this age increases the risk of infection. If his heart is on the wrong side then you will need a detailed family history, a chest X-ray, echocardiography and possibly a nasal mucosa biopsy. Grandma may never have heard of Kartagener syndrome, but she may well be wiser than you think!

CASE 15 NEAR DROWNING
A 10-year-old boy was seen floating at the bottom of the 10 foot deep end of the swimming baths during a school swimming lesson. He was spotted by an observant attendant, pulled out and successfully resuscitated. He is fully conscious on his arrival at the Emergency Department. You would organize

A   a skull X-ray to exclude a fracture
B   an EEG to exclude a fit
C   a cranial CT scan to exclude brain damage
D   an assessment by a clinical psychologist
E   that he did not swim for the next 3–6 months

CASE 16 CHEER FOR SOME, DEPRESSION FOR OTHERS
A 2-year-old inquisitive toddler is found by his mother with a bottle of dothiepin hydrochloride tablets. The top was off and some were missing. He had been born prematurely and required a prolonged period of intensive care followed by oxygen at home for broncho-pulmonary dysplasia. His mother has become depressed and the tablets had been prescribed for her. The mother rang her GP immediately who advised that she take him directly to hospital. The poison centre advise you that the tablets have the same side-effects as amitriptyline hydrochloride. You would

A   set up an intravenous line to give him plenty of fluid
B   administer a sedative
C   monitor his ECG for the next 12 hours
D   send the tablets for analysis
E   prescribe oral charcoal

CASE 17 DELAYED DIAGNOSIS
A 16-year-old man is considering his future. His 14-year-old sister has just died from cystic fibrosis confirmed at post-mortem. He has been treated since the age of 1 year for cystic fibrosis with chest physiotherapy and aggressive antibiotic therapy for respiratory infections. He is well grown and has good respiratory function. Three sweat tests at the age of 16 years show normal sodium and chloride secretion. It would be correct to tell him

A   he has recovered from cystic fibrosis
B   he is unlikely to be infertile
C   his life expectancy is normal
D   he does not have an increased risk of having children affected with cystic fibrosis
E   sweat tests are more reliable now than they were 15 years ago

(Answers overleaf)

CASE 15 **None**

To perform any of these investigations suggests that you have joined in the panic and over-reaction that follow such events. Everybody is bound to be over anxious. However, if there are no outward signs of injury and the boy is responding normally, a skull X-ray is unlikely to reveal that he banged his head. An EEG may be hard to resist. A positive finding does not mean that he had had a fit at the time; and a negative finding does not mean that he did not. Cranial CT scan and psychometry will only be indicated in those cases where neurological recovery is incomplete. He should be encouraged to swim again as soon as he feels able, provided adequate supervision is available.

CASE 16 **C   E**

The feared side-effects of amitriptylines are arrhythmias and heart block. The others include dry mouth, drowsiness, blurred vision and constipation. Amitriptyline can be toxic in small amounts and therefore activated charcoal may help in binding the drug in the stomach, thus reducing its absorption. Charcoal is likely to be most effective if it is given within 2 hours of ingestion.

CASE 17 **B   C**

Cystic fibrosis is an inherited condition, you either have it or you do not. Three normal sweat tests indicate that the initial diagnosis was incorrect. There is no reason to think that physiotherapy and an aggressive antibiotic therapy for respiratory infections renders the subject infertile or shortens life! He has a 50:50 chance of being a heterozygote for CF and therefore he has an increased risk of having an affected child. Sweat tests have always been reliable if properly performed but technical problems may give misleading results. That is why it is now the practice to perform three tests and review the diagnosis at regular intervals. Gene analysis should remove any uncertainties.

Misdiagnoses have occurred, and distressed and angry parents have turned to the courts because they believe they have been badly served.

CASE 18 HEART FAILURE

A 2-month-old boy presents with breathlessness which had developed over the last 6 hours, difficulty in feeding, and occasional regurgitation. On examination there are widespread coarse and fine crepitations. The heart rate is so rapid that the heart sounds are difficult to hear but they sound normal. The liver is 6 cm and the spleen 2 cm below the rib margin. Investigations which might help you determine whether the child is in heart failure include

A   examination of jugular vein pressure wave
B   percussion of the chest
C   looking for palmar sweating
D   palpation of peripheral pulses
E   a chest X-ray

CASE 19 AN ABRUPT COUGHING BOUT

A 6 year old had a coughing attack whilst in the playground at school and went blue in the face. He coughed so much he choked and vomited and then gradually improved. The school nurse decided she had better take him home, by which time he had fully recovered. Next day he was not himself, he developed a fever and intermittent cough. His family doctor gave an antibiotic but he remained unwell. A week later a chest X-ray revealed right middle lobe collapse and consolidation. It is still present 8 weeks later. You would

A   enquire if other children at the school had a similar illness
B   enquire what games they were playing in the school yard
C   perform a needle biopsy of the lung
D   ask for a bronchogram
E   arrange for bronchoscopy

CASE 20 WHOSE ANXIETY ARE YOU TREATING?

A 33-year-old mother of five children brings her youngest aged 2 years to hospital by taxi at 02.00 hours because he has croup. He has had it on and off for 3 days and she is exhausted. When he arrives he is fast asleep and not making a noise. On examination he is pink and there are no added sounds in his chest. You should

A   admit him to intensive care
B   arrange for laryngoscopy and elective intubation
C   send his mother home for a rest
D   give adrenaline by inhalation
E   give aminophylline intravenously

(Answers overleaf)

CASE 18 **B   D   E**
Distinguishing between severe bronchiolitis and heart failure can be very difficult. If in doubt treat for both. A key sign of heart failure is an enlarged liver; a key sign of severe bronchiolitis is an over inflated lung and a depressed liver. Percussion of the chest and a chest X-ray will help to resolve this issue. It is pointless to attempt to assess the jugular venous pressure in a distressed 2-month-old infant. A very rapid pulse occurs in both, but the absence of lower limb pulses would point to coarctation of the aorta as the cause of the heart failure. Sweating on the brow suggests heart failure; palmar sweat is under different control and is a marker of stress and would be expected in any acutely ill child.

CASE 19 **B   E**

The diagnosis is an inhaled foreign body until proved otherwise. A sudden onset of coughing, followed by a persistent area of collapse consolidation is very suggestive. He may have been playing some game with blow pipes and sucked when he should have blown and not realized where the pellet went. Bronchoscopy is the appropriate investigation and treatment.

CASE 20 **None**

Any experienced mother who brings her child to hospital in the middle of the night is very worried. There can be no question of sending him home again even if there is nothing abnormal to be found on examination. By the same token, it would be wrong to over-react and unnecessarily frighten the child. A gentle calm approach and care in a comfortable ward where the child can be properly observed is all that is required. There will be plenty of time to respond should the child deteriorate. If his mother is worried enough to bring him to hospital in the middle of the night she will probably want to stay. She should be offered a bed close to her child.

CASE 21 STOMACH PAINS
A 6-year-old boy suffers from recurrent right-sided abdominal pain. It comes on at any time and is always the same in character. There is no association with eating, bowel actions or micturation. It is occasionally followed by a headache. Mother had had a hysterectomy, and father suffers from peptic ulcers. It is appropriate to

A   prescribe paracetamol
B   send urine for microscopy
C   send stool for culture
D   arrange a barium meal
E   arrange renal ultrasound

CASE 22 DEHYDRATION
An infant aged 3 months weighing 5 kg is admitted to the Emergency Department with severe diarrhoea and vomiting. He is severely dehydrated, has deep rapid breathing and is unresponsive and twitching. You set up an intravenous infusion. It would be appropriate to give

A   normal saline, 20 ml per kg, immediately
B   5% glucose, 30–40 ml per kg, over the first 4 hours
C   8.4% sodium bicarbonate, 4 ml per kg, immediately
D   oral rehydration solution
E   an intravenous broad-spectrum antibiotic

CASE 23 A BOWEL DISORDER
A 10-year-old girl attends clinic complaining of unpleasant bluish red swellings around the anus and vulva. Enquiry reveals that she has tended to suffer from abdominal pains with occasional bouts of diarrhoea. On occasion there has been blood in the motion. Her height and weight fall below the 3rd centile. Investigations should include

A   protoscopy in outpatient clinic
B   stool culture
C   vaginal flora culture
D   barium meal
E   rectal biopsy

(Answers overleaf)

CASE 21 **A   B   E**

The critical feature of the history is the fact that the pain is *right sided*. The first and immediate responsibility of the doctor is to exclude a renal cause such as hydronephrosis. Whilst these studies are underway there is no reason why the child should not be given appropriate analgesia.

CASE 22 **A   C**

A rapid infusion of normal saline or plasma is needed to correct the reduced circulating volume. Glucose only solutions can cause cerebral oedema in hypernatraemic infants and should be avoided. 8.4% sodium bicarbonate is equivalent to 1 mmol of sodium bicarbonate in 1 ml (1000 mmol Na/l) and is very hypertonic. Cautious use of sodium bicarbonate is indicated if severe acidosis is present. In this infant profound acidosis is suggested by the deep rapid breathing. Oral rehydration therapy has achieved much in avoiding infants reaching this state, but once a child is semiconscious intravenous therapy is indicated. There is nothing in the information given to justify giving intravenous antibiotics.

CASE 23 **B   D   E**

The history and findings are very suggestive of Crohn disease. A protoscopy would be unpleasant and could only be considered at the time of an anaesthetic for diagnostic renal biopsy. A stool culture is non-invasive and should be done to exclude superadded infections. A barium meal will reveal the extent of the lesion in the small bowel. A barium enema will show the extent of large bowel involvement. In the light of the clinical features it might be difficult to justify a rectal biopsy.

CASE 24 TIME TO TAKE A STAND
A baby is born vaginally at term weighing 4.1 kg. He cries at birth
and behaves well and is normal on routine neonatal examination. His
mother dislikes hospital and elects to take him home at 6 hours of
age. Three days later, on a Sunday evening, he is reluctant to feed
and his mother does not like the look of him. She calls the doctor
who notes that the infant's breathing is rapid and the child appears
cyanosed. When he arrives in A&E you find an ill infant with a rapid
pulse and distressed breathing. You would be correct to hold the
view that

A   the failure to detect any abnormality on examination at birth makes
    a significant congenital heart defect unlikely
B   it is essential that the infant's cardiac state is investigated that
    evening
C   blood cultures should be taken and intravenous antibiotics
    commenced
D   if his mother wishes to take her child home that evening, he should
    be held in hospital against her wishes
E   his collapse would have been avoided if he had stayed in hospital
    from birth

CASE 25 STRIKING SWELLINGS
A boy aged 3 years presents with vague stomach pain and swelling
on the face, scrotum and penis. Examination reveals leg oedema and
ascites. The urine contains protein but not blood or cells. The parents
are naturally anxious. You would be correct in advising them that

A   provided the child eats an adequate protein diet the problem will
    not recur
B   it is probable that he will need a renal transplant before he reaches
    adulthood
C   in all probability his condition can be controlled by corticosteroids
D   they must learn to measure his blood pressure
E   they must learn to test his urine and record it in a book

(Answers overleaf)

CASE 24 **B C D**

It is not uncommon for a severe congenital heart defect to present towards the end of the first week of life. If whole body or selective imaging becomes part of the routine assessment of newborn infants, most heart lesions will be detected at birth before problems develop. In the meantime, they should be sought in any infant who presents with poor feeding and cyanotic episodes. Very occasionally the child's collapse is precipitated by closure of the ductus arteriosus and the infusion of drugs to keep it open may be life saving, therefore the diagnosis is an emergency.

Bacterial infection is another possibility and antibiotic therapy should not be delayed until culture results are available.

Parents sometimes have real though irrational fear of hospitals. In times of stress they may not always behave sensibly. Your duty is to put the child's interests first, to avoid conflict, to help the parents, but in the final analysis resist their intention to take their child home, by obtaining the appropriate court orders if necessary.

Babies with severe infections or heart defects collapse like this in hospital, and there is no reason to think that being at home increased the risk. One would hope that there would have been less delay before the problem was recognized and addressed.

CASE 25 **C E**

The management and prognosis of nephrotic syndrome are very different in children compared with adults. The vast majority respond to corticosteroid therapy and, despite frequent relapses during childhood, often grow out of it by late adolescence. The aim of management is to make them as independent of hospital as possible. For this they need to be able to test the urine for protein, and to learn to judge when corticosteroids are necessary.

CASE 26 EXCESSIVE BRUISING
A 6-year-old boy presents with a florid bruise in the forehead following a minor bump. On inspection he has a fine petechial rash of which both he and his parents were unaware. His sister suffered from rubella 5 weeks ago. There are enlarged lymph nodes in the upper cervical group but none elsewhere. The liver is not enlarged, and the tip of the spleen can just be palpated. With this history it is probable that investigation will show

A   platelet count below 5 × 10⁹/l
B   spherocytes in the peripheral blood film
C   marked lymphocytosis with occasional abnormal cells
D   meningococci growing from a blood culture
E   increased megakaryoctes in a bone marrow aspirate

CASE 27 A SUSPICIOUS MASS
A mother, whilst bathing her 9-month-old baby, feels a hard mass in her abdomen. The examining doctor notes that the mass crosses the midline and merges with the liver. An abdominal X-ray shows diffuse speckled calcification. The parents should be told that

A   their child has cancer
B   survival and resolution occurs in nearly 50%
C   there have been considerable improvements in survival rates as new therapies have been introduced
D   the course of the disease can be monitored by testing the urine
E   scoliosis is one of the complications of treatment

CASE 28 COLD HANDS AND FEET
A mother of five brings her youngest, aged 18 months, to clinic because his hands and feet are invariably cold, and either blue or blotchy blue and red. The baby is not breathless and is said to feed well. On examination, the infant is underweight, his heart sounds are normal, the peripheral pulses are full and the hands and feet look unusually small. You would

A   arrange for a chest X-ray
B   make enquiry from the family's Health Visitor about his feeding pattern
C   consider the diagnosis of Raynaud phenomenon
D   recommend the use of mittens and thick socks
E   enquire about domestic arrangements

(Answers overleaf)

CASE 26 **A E**

The probable diagnosis is idiopathic or immune thrombocytopenia. Leukaemia has to be considered and positively excluded but it is unusual for it to present with purpura alone. Meningococcal septicaemia and Henoch Schönlein purpura give a purpuric rash due to a vasculitis; they do not cause an increased bleeding tendency.

CASE 27 **A B E**

The plain abdominal X-ray may be highly suggestive of neuroblastoma. Abdominal CT scans and urinary vanilmandelic acid (VMA) will confirm the diagnosis and make the distinction from nephroblastoma. The parents must be given an honest account of modern thoughts on management and survival. Survival is greater in children under the age of 2 years. Sadly, modern aggressive treatment regimens have not had much impact on malignancy. Urinary VMA is not a reliable guide with which to monitor the success of treatment. Disturbed spinal growth is a potential long-term problem after radiotherapy.

CASE 28 **B E**

The deprivation syndrome sometimes produces some remarkable and inexplicable findings both on history and examination. Why such children develop cold, blue/red, small hands and feet is unknown.

CASE 29 THIRST AND ABDOMINAL PAIN
A 5-year-old boy previously admitted to a surgical ward as an emergency with abdominal pain is later the same evening referred to the medical team. He is breathless and his breath smells sweet. His mother has brought in a bottle of orange juice because in the last week or so he has repeatedly asked for drinks. You would

A   arrange for a chest X-ray to exclude pneumonia
B   arrange for an intravenous pyelogram
C   send his urine for culture and sensitivity
D   take blood for pH measurement
E   give intravenous normal saline with added potassium chloride

CASE 30 RED LUMPS
A 12-year-old boy develops red painful lumps over his shins varying in maximum diameter from 0.5 to 10 cm. He has a high temperature and pain on moving his right knee and left elbow. The ESR is raised. It would be important to

A   measure antistreptolysin titre
B   perform tuberculin 1:1000 skin test (Mantoux)
C   record ECG
D   measure antinuclear antibodies
E   arrange a chest X-ray

CASE 31 SEXUAL ABUSE
An anxious social worker brings a 5-year-old girl to be examined because she told her nursery teacher that her mother's boyfriend 'had pushed his thing up inside her'. You examine her and consider the following consistent with her story

A   finger tip bruising of the waist
B   multiple anal fissures
C   labial fusion
D   anal dilatation on buttock separation
E   anal warts

CASE 32 RASH AND FITS
A 4-year-old boy is admitted after having a fit. He is still drowsy but general examination is normal, except for a blotchy petechial rash over the lower half of his body. Your prelimary investigations would include

A   full blood count and film analysis
B   bone marrow aspiration
C   cranial CT scan
D   culture of blood
E   lumbar puncture

(Answers overleaf)

CASE 29 **D   E**

Fewer than 10% of new diabetics now present with ketoacidosis, but it remains an important diagnosis in a child presenting with abdominal pain. Prompt diagnosis is straightforward based on a random blood glucose measurement, glycosuria, and ketonuria. Other investigations allow estimation of the severity of acidosis, fluid and electrolyte imbalance.

CASE 30 **A   C   E**

Erythema nodosum may be associated with streptococcal reactions (ASO titre), rheumatic fever (ECG), tuberculosis (with hypersensitivity use only 1:10 000 tuberculin) and sarcoid (chest X-ray). In the UK the majority of causes are innocent and often difficult to define.

CASE 31 **A   B   C   D   E**

These signs are all consistent with some form of sexual abuse but they may also have other explanations. In themselves they do not establish that abuse has taken place. They have to be reviewed in the light of the circumstances revealed by careful skilled evaluation of the child and her environment.

CASE 32 **A   D   E**

The likely diagnosis is meningococcal septicaemia and meningitis. A cerebral bleed due to idiopathic thrombocytopenia is a rare but important alternative. The immediate priorities are confirmation with blood and cerebrospinal fluid culture, intravenous antibiotics and correction of circulatory collapse. While benzylpenicillin is appropriate for meningococcal infection, it should be remembered that *Haemophilus influenzae* and other pathogens can occasionally cause septicaemia accompanied by purpura.

CASE 33 VISUAL DEFECT
An infant aged 4 months old who had been born at 26 weeks gestation is found on examination in follow-up clinic not to be fixing upon the examiner's face. This might be because

A an infant at this age does not fix on a strange face
B the infant is too young to fix upon a face
C the infant is myopic
D the infant had been given gentamycin
E the infant has retinopathy of prematurity

CASE 34 SLOW PROGRESS
A young girl aged 18 months was taken by her mother to her family doctor because she appeared to be slow in her movements. Apparently medical examination did not reveal anything unusual, and she was reassured. When she was 21 months old she still had not got any teeth. The orthodontist suspected the diagnosis. Confirmatory evidence might be obtained by

A measuring serum bilirubin levels
B performing a knee jerk
C testing visual fields
D recording sleeping pulse rate
E measuring the level of thyroid stimulating hormone in the blood

CASE 35 QUESTIONS TO ANSWER
Parents bring their overweight 3-year-old child to see you in clinic. He has cerebral palsy and fits. The notes tell you that he suffered from enterobacter meningitis soon after birth and has had a shunt put in place for hydrocephalus. The parents have made a list of the questions they want to ask you. Would they be right to conclude that

A they were referred to their dietitian because they needed advice on how to feed their child and not because their son had a health problem
B they should give permission for him to have the measles vaccine
C the tests for liver function which he had last month, after he had been commenced on sodium valproate, were to determine whether he also had underlying liver disease
D he is more likely to have fits when he is sleepy
E an increased dose of sodium valproate makes him sleepy

(Answers overleaf)

CASE 33 **E**

Whilst as many as 50% of infants born at 26 weeks gestation develop some degree of retinopathy of prematurity (retrolental fibroplasia), only a very small percentage progress to irreversible scarring and blindness. The reasons for this are unknown. Many factors are now thought to contribute to the development of the lesions of which oxygen is only one. The lesions frequently develop despite close monitoring of arterial oxygen concentrations.

CASE 34 **B E**

Congenital hypothyroidism may manifest in early infancy (prolonged jaundice and poor feeding) or later in childhood (growth failure, developmental delay and constipation). The unreliable results of clinical detection justified the introduction of thyroid screening programmes. These have proved highly successful and have substantially reduced the resulting problem of mental handicap.

CASE 35 **A B D E**

There would be little point in advising this young man about his diet. Nonetheless it is good practice to explain to the parents why you are referring them to another colleague for professional advice. It is important that he has all the protection that the vaccination programme offers. In children with brain damage the effects of anticonvulsants are hard to predict. It is as well to listen to what the parents say and accept their assessment unless you have very good reason for knowing that they are mistaken. The liver function was tested to see if the drug was affecting the liver, not to seek additional underlying disease.

CASE 36 IT MAKES HIM SICK
A distraught mother brings her 10-month-old boy to hospital at her GP's request. For 6 weeks he has had diarrhoea and vomiting on and off. In the last 2 days he has vomited everything he has swallowed. She thinks he has lost weight. On taking a dietary history you learn that he has always been a difficult feeder. When he was 4 weeks old, his mother was advised to try to feed him on an infant formula based on soybean protein. He was weaned on to normal foods at 4 months of age. Over the last 6 weeks he has taken dilute milk and water and electrolyte solutions only. You start him on a formula containing predigested protein and medium chain triglycerides (MCT). The following are facts on which you could rely

A   a soy-based formula does not contain lactose
B   soy-based feeds are made with vegetable oils and therefore have a lower content of essential fatty acids than cow's milk based formula
C   protein sensitivity will not develop if cow's milk is excluded in all forms from his diet
D   his dietary history makes gluten enteropathy unlikely
E   MCT absorption is dependent on bile acid secretion

CASE 37 CONFUSED AND FITTING
A 2-year-old girl of mixed parentage begins to behave oddly and no longer appears to recognize her parents. She develops a fever and has a fit. She has had afebrile convulsions before. Next day she is reluctant to stand and says very little. She has had middle ear infection in the past and is on the waiting list for insertion of grommets. On the third day of the illness she has three fits in succession at home and is brought to hospital. She has another fit as soon as she is admitted to the ward and then falls asleep. On neurological examination there are no localizing signs. The eyes move normally and there is no papilloedema. The CT scan is normal, and the cerebrospinal fluid is clear without increased cells. You would advise her parents that

A   her encephalopathic illness is a complication of febrile fits
B   given the nature of the presentation it is likely that she will be left with permanent brain damage
C   she does not have a brain tumour
D   she does not have meningitis
E   the most likely cause is a viral infection

(Answers overleaf)

CASE 36 **A   D**

Soy-based feeds do not contain lactose and they are useful in the treatment of lactose intolerance. Vegetable oils do contain essential fatty acids but only traces of the polyunsaturated fats. Some children develop sensitivity to soy protein. Legally it is not acceptable to describe soy-based formulae as milk even though they are 'complete feeds'. There is no milk in them. Continued vomiting with recent deterioration whilst he has been fed with milk and clear fluids only, make gluten sensitivity most unlikely. MCT are formed of fatty acids of mid-chain length (C8–C12); they are more water soluble, they do not need bile acids for absorption and are absorbed into the portal vein.

CASE 37 **C   D   E**

Febrile fits by definition are 'uncomplicated'. In the UK National Encephalopathy Study which was established to determine whether the whooping cough vaccine was responsible for brain damaging illness, over 1000 episodes of encephalopathic illness were reported in little over a year. The vast majority of those who did not have brain damage before the event recovered fully. With improving diagnostic techniques more and more encephalopathic episodes are being found to be due to viral illness.

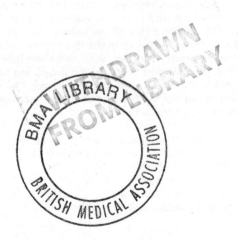

CASE 38 YELLOW ALERT
A GP refers a breastfed Asian 6-week-old infant to clinic because of persisting jaundice. The mother is confident that his urine is pale and clear. As far as she is concerned his stools are normal in colour, consistency and smell. He feeds happily and appears to be a contented child. She wants to have him circumcised next week for religious reasons. You would

A   measure the conjugated and unconjugated levels of bilirubin in the *mother's* and infant's blood
B   advise her that in all probability the jaundice is due to breastfeeding
C   reassure her that the moderate jaundice itself does not cause lasting harm
D   examine the child's eyes for cataract formation
E   advise her to delay the operation for circumcision until you have the results of your investigations

CASE 39 AN ETHICAL DILEMMA
A 10-month-old girl with a rare chromosome abnormality of uncertain prognosis is admitted with a body temperature of 34°C. Her parents appear loving and deeply concerned. The child has very limited spontaneous movements and is subject to fits. It is proper to

A   look for an underlying infection and give antibiotics whilst awaiting the results of the investigation
B   advise the parents that hypothermia commonly precedes death in infancy
C   withdraw anticonvulsant therapy
D   place the parents under covert surveillance
E   ensure that she is always well wrapped up whilst she is in hospital and counsel the parents to do likewise when they take her home

(Answers overleaf)

CASE 38 **B   C   D   E**

From the history it is unlikely that this infant has underlying liver disease or that his jaundice is due to an inherited metabolic disorder. However, it is good practice to look into the eyes for obvious cataract formation and it would be important to exclude liver disease before subjecting him to a surgical procedure which might be complicated by bleeding.

CASE 39 **A**

Until you have a full understanding of the child's condition and her parents' wishes, she must be treated like any other. Care must be taken to keep her in circumstances which allow her to have a normal body temperature. High temperatures are more immediately dangerous than low temperatures.

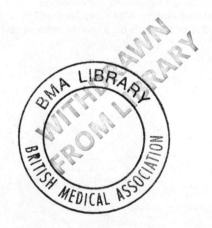